A
CONCISE
DICTIONARY
OF
MEDICINE

A CONCISE
DICTIONARY
OF MEDICINE

by M.W. Martin

jD | JONATHAN DAVID PUBLISHERS, INC.
MIDDLE VILLAGE, N.Y. 11379

A CONCISE DICTIONARY OF MEDICINE

by

M.W. Martin

Copyright © 1975

by

Jonathan David Publishers

Jonathan David Publishers
68-22 Eliot Avenue
Middle Village, New York 11379

Library of Congress Cataloging in Publication Data

Martin, M.W.
  A concise dictionary of medicine.

  1. Medicine—Dictionaries. I. Title.
[DNLM: 1. Dictionaries, Medical. W13 M382c]
R121.M44   610'.3   74-23215
ISBN 0-8246-0193-9

Printed in the United States of America

abasia Inability to walk.

abatement The lessening or moderation of intensity of pain or of symptoms of a disease.

abdomen A body cavity occupying the space between the diaphragm and the pelvis.

abdominal angina An attack of severe abdominal pain, commonly occurring after eating.

abdominohysterectomy The removal of the uterus (womb) through an abdominal incision.

abducent nerve The sixth cranial nerve. It regulates the muscles which rotate the eyeball away from the midline of the body.

abductor A muscle which draws or pulls a body part away from its midline, or axis; the opposite of adductor.

aberration Anything abnormal.

abiosis Nonliving; the absence of life.

abirritant A substance, such as a cream or powder, that relieves irritation.

ablactation The end of the period when a breast gives milk.

ablation The removal of any harmful or abnormal growth from the body.

ablepharia A total or partial absence of the eyelids caused by a birth defect.

ablepsia Blindness.

abort To miscarry.

abortifacient A drug used to induce an abortion.

abortion The purposeful expulsion of a nonliving embryo or fetus from the womb.

abrade To scrape away, as to abrade the skin.

abrasion A scrape or scratch of the skin.

abreaction In psychoanalysis, the mental process by which repressed, unconscious and forgotten memories and experiences are brought to consciousness.

abscess A localized accumulation of pus.

abstraction Absent-mindedness. Preoccupation.

abulia Inability to make decisions.

a.c. Abbreviation for "before meals," used in writing prescriptions.

acalculia The inability to learn or do even the simplest arithmetical problems.

acampsia Inflexibility or rigidity of a joint.

acanthesthesia An abnormal feeling of being pricked with needles.

acanthoma A tumor of the skin.

acanthosis A skin condition marked by thickening warty growths.

acapnia Complete absence of carbon dioxide from the blood.

acatamathesia The inability to understand conversation.

acataphasia The loss of the ability to speak in orderly sentences.

acathexia The inability to retain bodily secretions and excretions.

accomodation Adjustment of the eye to new surroundings, as to the dark, when coming in from daylight.

accouchement Confinement for delivery; childbirth.

accretion Growth by the adding of identical substance to the outside of a structure; an accumulation.

acenesthesia Lack or loss of the normal sensation of one's own body.

aceratosis Absence of nails on extremities.

acetabulectomy The surgical removal of the acetabulum.

acetabuloplasty Any operation aimed to reshape the acetabulum to fit the head of the thigh bone.

acetabulum The cup-shaped cavity in the hip bone into which the rounded head of the thigh bone fits to form a ball-and-socket joint.

acetic acid The acid of vinegar occasionally used, when diluted, as a counterirritant.

6

acetone A chemical substance often found in large quantities in persons with diabetes.

acetonemia The presence of acetone in the blood in relatively large amounts.

acetonuria Excess acetone in the urine.

acetylcholine A chemical substance, produced within the body aiding the transmission of nerve impulses.

acetylsalicylic acid Aspirin.

Achilles tendon The tendon that binds muscles in the calf of the leg to the heel bone.

ACH index An index of nutrition based on measurements of arm girth, chest depth, and hip width.

achlorhydria The absence of hydrochloric acid from the gastric juices of the stomach.

achluophobia Morbid fear of darkness.

achromatopsia Total color blindness due to disease or injury of the retina or optic nerve.

Achromycin A trademark for tetracycline, an antibiotic drug.

achylia gastrica The lack of hydrochloride acid and rennin in gastric juices.

acidosis Acid intoxication due to faulty metabolism and elimination of acid chemicals.

acidulate To make acid; to render sour.

aciduria Acid urine.

acne A condition of the skin common in adolescence and young adulthood, characterized by an eruption of pimples and blackheads.

aconuresis Involuntary urination.

acoria A sensation of hunger not even relieved by a large meal.

acoustic nerve The eighth cranial nerve, which supplies the ear.

acousticophobia Morbid fear of sounds.

acroagnosis The lack of sensation in a limb.

acroarthritis Arthritis of the arms or legs.

acrocephaly A pointed head; a birth defect.

acrocyanosis Cold and blue hands and feet.

7

acrodermatitis Any inflammation of the hands, arms, teet or legs.

acroedema Persisting swelling of the arms and feet.

acrogeria Wrinkling of the skin of the hands and feet, caused by premature aging.

acrohyperhidrosis The excessive sweating of the hands, feet, or both.

acromania Madness.

acromegaly A chronic disease, usually of middle life, due to excessive function of the pituitary gland.

acronyx An ingrown nail.

acropathy An abnormal condition of the arms or legs.

acrophobia Morbid dread of great heights.

acrylics Plastic materials used in making false teeth, dentures and lenses.

ACTH The abbreviation for the adrenocorticotropic hormone.

actinomycosis "Lumpy jaw;" a fungus infection of men and cattle.

activated charcoal A medicinal grade of charcoal used to absorb poisons, and as an antidote against various poisons.

acuity Clearness (in vision or hearing).

acupuncture Needling in order to relieve pain. It is used chiefly in Chinese medicine.

acute Sharp, severe, sudden, rapid; not chronic.

acute abdomen A condition within the abdomen, requiring prompt surgery.

acute yellow atrophy Rapid, massive destruction of the liver, usually as a result of viral hepatitis.

acyanopsia Inability to see blue colors.

adacrya Absence of tears.

adactylia The absence of fingers, toes, or both. A birth deformity.

Adams-Stokes disease (or **syndrome**) Repeated fainting (unconsciousness), sometimes with convulsions.

Addison's disease A serious illness caused by insufficiency or non-function of the adrenal glands.

adduct To move a part of the body, usually an arm or leg, toward the midline.

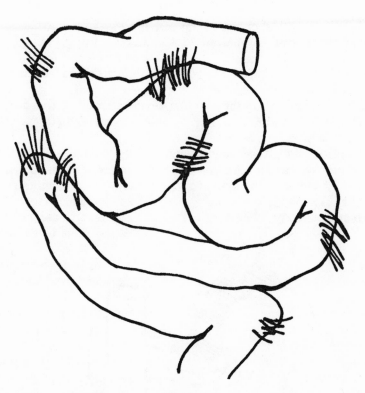

Adhesions.

adenectomy The surgical removal of a gland.

adenitis The inflammation of a gland, usually a lymph gland.

adenocarcinoma Cancer originating in a gland.

adenocellulitis Inflammation of a gland and the surrounding tissue.

adenofibroma A combined benign tumor consisting of gland tissue and fibrous tissue most often seen in the breast or in the uterus.

adenoid Lymph gland located in the throat behind the nose.

adenoidectomy The surgical removal of the adenoids.

adenoma A benign tumor in which the cell arrangement resembles a gland-like structure.

adenopathy Any glandular disease, especially one marked by swelling and enlargement of lymph glands.

adenosarcoma A malignant tumor containing both gland and connective tissue.

adenotonsillectomy The surgical removal of the tonsils and adenoids.

ADH Abbreviation for *antidiuretic hormone.*

adhesion An abnormal fibrous union of one organ (or part) to another.

adiaphoresis Absence of sweat.

adiposis dolorosa A disease in which there are areas of painful fat beneath the skin occurring mainly in women during the menopause.

adrenalectomy The surgical removal of the adrenal glands.

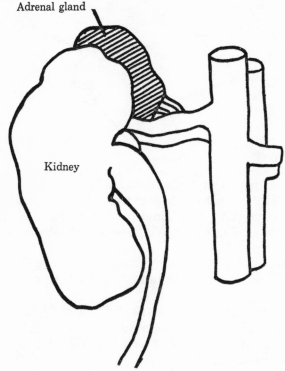

Adrenal gland

Kidney

The adrenal gland.

adrenal glands Two glands in the abdomen which produce adrenalin and other hormones.

adrenalin One of the hormones produced by the adrenal glands.

adrenalitis An inflammation of the adrenal glands.

adrenocorticotropic hormone (ACTH) A hormone produced by the pituitary gland which influences the function of the adrenal and other glands of the body.

adynamia The loss of vital strength or muscular power; weakness.

Aedes aegypti The mosquito which transmits yellow fever and dengue fever.

aeroembolism Decompression sickness.

aerogram An X-ray picture of an organ inflated with air.

aero-otitis An inflammation of the middle ear caused by changes in altitude in airplane flights.

aerophagia Air swallowing, sometimes hysterical.

aerophobia A morbid fear of drafts or of fresh air.

aeroscope An instrument for the examination of air dust and for estimating the purity of the air.

aerotherapeutics A mode of treating disease by varying the pressure or the composition of the air breathed.

afebrile Without fever.

affinity Inherent attraction and relationship.

affusion The pouring of water upon a part or upon the body, as in fever, to reduce temperature and calm nervous symptoms.

afterbirth The placenta and membranes which are discharged from the vagina following the birth of a child.

agalorrhea The stoppage of milk flow from the breast.

agammaglobulinemia The lack of necessary gamma globulin in the blood.

agar An extract of seaweed often used as a culture medium for growing bacteria in the laboratory.

aglutition Difficulty in swallowing.

agnosia The total or partial loss of ability to recognize persons or things.

agonad A person without sex glands.

11

agoraphobia Fear of open spaces.

agranulocytosis A rare but often fatal disease in which there are too few white blood cells in the blood.

agraphia The loss of the ability to write, due to a brain disease.

agromania An abnormal desire to live in the open country or in isolation.

agrypnia Insomnia.

ague An old word commonly associated with the chills and fevers produced by malaria.

AHF Abbreviation for *antihemophilic factor*; now called *factor VIII*.

AHG Abbreviation for *antihemophilic globulin*; now called *factor VIII*.

aichmophobia The dread of sharp or pointed objects, or of being touched by them or by a finger.

ailurophobia Morbid fear of cats.

air passages The nares, nasal cavities, pharynx, mouth, larynx, trachea, and bronchial tubes.

akinesia Immobility.

alalia Loss of speech.

Albamycin A trademark for *novobiocin*, an antibiotic particularly effective against staphylococcal infections.

albino An individual lacking pigment in the skin, hair, and eyes.

albumin A common and important protein component of living animal tissues.

aldosterone A hormone produced by the adrenal gland.

alexia Loss of the ability to understand the meaning of printed or written words.

alienist A psychiatrist.

alimentary canal The food tract, beginning with the mouth and extending for 20 to 25 feet to the anus; also called the *gastrointestinal tract*.

alimentation Feeding.

alkalosis The excess of alkali in the fluids and tissues of the body; usually too much bicarbonate in the blood. The opposite of acidosis.

allergen Any substance which is able to cause an allergic condition.

allergist A physician who specializes in the diagnosis and treatment of allergic diseases.

allergy A condition whereby a person reacts abnormally to a specific substance.

allopathy A method of medical treatment using remedies that produce effects upon the body differing from those produced by disease.

alloplasty Any plastic operation in which material from outside the human body, such as a metal, plastic, or bone, is used.

allopurinol A drug which suppresses the body's production of uric acid; used in the treatment of gout.

aloe An herb used in chronic constipation for its stimulating effect on the large intestine.

alopecia Loss of hair.

alum A substance which produces constriction.

aluminum hydroxide gel An antacid, often prescribed for stomach ulcers.

alusia Hallucination.

alveoli The small air cells of the lung.

alveolitis An inflammation of tooth sockets and gums; a frequent complication after tooth extraction.

alysmus The anxiety and restlessness which accompany physical disease.

amalgam A combination of mercury with other metals used for restoring teeth and for making dental dies.

amaurosis Blindness due to nervous disorders.

ambisexual The feelings and behavior which are neither strictly masculine nor feminine, but common to both sexes.

ambivert A personality type intermediate between extrovert and introvert.

ambrosia Ragweed.

ambulatory Able to walk by oneself.

ameba A tiny one-celled animal.

amebiasis An infection caused by an organism called *endameba histolytica* which lodges in the bowels.

amebic dysentery Severe amebiasis, characterized by diarrhea (often containing mucus and blood), abdominal cramp-- ing, and fever.

amenorrhea The absence or stoppage of menstruation; a "missed period."

amentia Subnormal mental development.

ametria Absence of the uterus; a birth deformity.

ametropia Poor vision due to failure of the image to focus upon the retina.

amino acids A large group of chemical compounds, containing nitrogen, that are the building blocks of protein.

ammonia A strong and rapidly acting stimulant used in smelling salts for relief in cases of fainting or exhaustion.

amnesia Loss of memory.

amnion The sac surrounding the embryo in the uterus.

amniotic fluid The fluid surrounding the embryo in the womb.

amphetamine A drug which stimulates the central nervous system; a common ingredient in "pep pills."

ampicillin A powerful antibiotic drug similar in structure and actions to penicillin.

ampule A sealed glass tube containing a measured amount of medication.

amputation The removal of a limb, in whole or in part.

amyl nitrite A drug which causes blood vessels to dilate promptly.

amyotonia Absence of muscle tone.

amyotrophic diseases Disorders that cause degeneration of muscle.

amyotrophic lateral sclerosis Muscle degeneration and spinal cord degeneration.

amyotrophy Muscular atrophy.

anabolism The process by which food is converted into living tissue.

anacidity The complete absence of hydrochloric acid in the stomach. Also termed *achlorhydria*.

anaclitic depression A sudden and striking impairment of an infant's physical, social and intellectual development.

anacousia Complete deafness.

anal erotic   Sexual drives and desires related to the anal zone.

analeptic drugs   Medications used to stimulate convalescence.

analgesia   Insensibility to pain without loss of consciousness.

analgesic   Pain-killer.

anaphia   A defective sense of touch, abnormal sensitivity to touch.

anaphoresis   The malfunction of the sweat glands.

anaphylaxis   The opposite of immunity.

anasarca   An accumulation of fluid in tissues.

anastomosis   The joining together of two or more hollow organs.

anatomy   The science of the structure of the body.

ancillary   Secondary.

ancylostoma   Hookworm; the parasite causing hookworm disease.

Andersen's syndrome   Cystic fibrosis of the pancreas.

andriatrics   A branch of medicine dealing with disorders peculiar to men, especially of the genitalia.

androgen   A male hormone that produces and controls the secondary male sex characteristics, such as the beard, muscles, deep voice, etc.

androsterone   One of the male sex hormones.

anemia   A disease of the blood characterized by an insufficiency of red blood cells, either in quality or quantity.

  anemia, aplastic   Anemia due to bone marrow defects and degenerative changes.

  anemia, hemolytic   Anemia caused by an agent which destroys red blood cells, such as in a snake bite.

  anemia, hemorrhagic   Anemia caused by direct or hidden bleeding.

  anemia lymphatica   Hodgkin's disease.

  anemia neonatorum   Anemia of the newborn.

  anemia, pernicious   A common and serious type of anemia associated with lack of hydrochloric acid in the stomach juices and nervous disorders.

  anemia, secondary   An anemia which is due to some other disease, such as cancer, tuberculosis, etc.

anemia, sickle cell A type of anemia occurring mainly among Negroes or dark-skinned people. It takes its name from the characteristic sickle shape of the red blood cells.

anergy Lack of energy.

anesthetic agent A drug which induces anesthesia.

anesthesia The absence of pain sensation, with or without loss of consciousness.

anesthesiologist A physician who specializes in the administration of anesthesia.

aneurysm Dilatation of an artery or vein caused when a weak spot occurs in the wall.

aneurysmectomy The surgical removal of an aneurysm.

aneuthanasia A painful or difficult death.

angina Any repeated, suffocating pain.

angina pectoris Pain in the chest, a symptom which accompanies any interference with blood supply or oxygenation of the heart muscle. It is a form of heart disease.

angio- Pertaining to a lymph or blood vessel.

angioblastoma A malignant tumor composed of blood vessel tissues.

angiocardiography X-ray visualization of the chambers of the heart and the large blood vessels entering or leaving the heart.

angiography X-ray of blood vessels after injections of a radiopaque substance to show their outlines.

angioma A tumor composed of lymph and blood vessels.

angiomalacia Softening of the blood vessels.

angioneurotic edema Swelling of the skin, mucous membranes, or internal organs.

angiopathy Any disease of the vascular system.

angioplasty Plastic surgery of injured or diseased veins or arteries.

angiorrhaphy Surgical repair of a blood vessel.

angiosarcoma A malignant tumor originating from blood vessels.

angiosclerosis Hardening and thickening of the walls of the blood vessels.

angiospasm Prolonged, strong contraction of a blood vessel.

angiotomy   Incision into a blood vessel.

angophrasia   A halting, choking, and drawling type of speech occurring in general paralysis.

anhidrosis   Failure of sweat gland function.

aniline   A coal tar derivative.

ankylosis   A stiff joint, resulting from disease or deliberate operation to immobilize the joint.

ankylodactylia   A deformity resulting from the adhesion of fingers or toes to one another.

ankyloglossia   Tongue-tie.

ankylostoma   Lockjaw.

annular   Ring-shaped.

anodyne   Any medication that relieves pain.

Anopheles   A genus of mosquitoes which transmits malaria and other diseases such as yellow fever.

anoplasty   Plastic surgery or repair of the anus.

anorchidism   Absence of the testicles.

anorexia nervosa   A hysterical aversion toward food.

anorgasmy   The failure or inability to reach a climax during sexual intercourse.

anosmia   Complete loss of the sense of smell.

anovulatory drugs   Those medications which inhibit and prevent ovulation.

anoxemia   Too little oxygen in the blood.

anoxia   Lack of oxygen.

Antabuse   Trademark for *disulfiram,* a drug used in the treatment of alcoholism.

antacid   A substance that relieves acidity and neutralizes acids.

antagonist   A drug which neutralizes the effect of another drug.

antenatal   Occurring before birth.

antepartum   Occurring before childbirth.

anteverted   Tipped forward, especially as an anteverted uterus.

anthelmintic   Any drug that destroys or chases worms from the body.

anthrax   A serious infectious disease in sheep or cattle, which is sometimes transmitted to humans.

anthypnotic   An agent that tends to keep one awake.

antibiotics   Substances produced during the growth of molds or bacteria which inhibit or kill other bacteria that cause disease.

antibody   A substance—natural or artificial—which is capable of producing a specific immunity to a specific germ or virus.

anticarcinogen   Any substance used in an attempt to block cancer development.

anticoagulant   A substance which prevents blood clotting.

anticonvulsant   A medication that prevents or stops convulsions.

antidote   A substance which counteracts a poison.

antigen   Any substance which produces antibodies.

antihistamine drugs   Synthetic substances used to alleviate allergic conditions.

antipruritic   A medication that relieves or prevents itching.

antipyretic   Anything that reduces or prevents fever.

antiseptic   An agent which inhibits or destroys bacteria.

antitoxin   A substance which neutralizes the effects of a poison released by bacteria.

antrostomy   Surgical opening of an antrum for drainage.

antrum   A cavity or hollow space, usually within a bone. It most frequently refers to the maxillary sinus in the upper jaw.

anuria   Inability to void urine. Also called **anuresis**.

anus   The end of the rectum near the buttocks.

aorta   The large artery originating from the left ventricle of the heart which distributes blood to all parts of the body.

aortitis   An inflammation of the aorta.

aortogram   X-ray of the aorta after injection of a radiopaque substance.

APC   A commonly prescribed capsule or tablet for headaches, colds, etc.

aperient   A mild laxative.

aphagia   Inability to swallow.

aphakia   Absence of the lens of the eye.

aphasia   The loss of speech

18

aphonia   Loss of speech because of hysteria or due to a condition located in the larynx.

aphrodisiac   Anything that stimulates sexual desire.

aphrodisiomania   Exaggerates sexual interest and excitement.

aphtha   A white painful mouth ulcer of unknown cause.

aphthous stomatitis   Inflammation of the mouth mucosa, characterized by the presence of small, painful blisters.

aphthous ulcer   Sore of the mouth.

apical abscess   An infection at the root of a tooth.

aplasia   Failure of a part or an organ to develop.

apnea   The cessation of breathing.

apocrine glands   Sweat glands.

apoplexy   A stroke resulting from a hemorrhage into the brain and marked by unconsciousness usually followed by paralysis of various parts of the body.

appendectomy   The surgical removal of the appendix.

appendicitis   Inflammation of the appendix.

appendix   A finger-shaped sac three to six inches long which projects from the large bowel, in the lower right quarter of the abdomen.

approach   A surgical term referring to the technique of getting to an organ.

apraxia   Inability to coordinate one's muscles and movements, usually due to a brain condition.

apyrexia   Absence of fever.

aqueous   Watery.

arachnoid   A membrane covering the brain and spinal cord.

arachnoidism   Poisoning by a spider bite.

arachnoiditis   Inflammation of the arachnoid membrane.

arciform   Shaped like a bow.

areflexia   Lack of reflexes.

areola   A rim around a central area, such as the mammary areola (the pigmented ring surrounding the nipple).

ariboflavinosis   Too little of the vitamin riboflavin in the diet.

Arlidin   Trademark for *nylidrin,* a drug helpful in producing blood vessel dilatation and combatting arterial spasm.

arrythmia Out of time; **cardiac arrhythmia** off-beat heart.

arteriectomy The surgical removal of an artery or portion of an artery.

arteriography X-ray of arteries.

arteriole A small artery.

arteriosclerosis Hardening of the arteries.

arteritis Inflammation of an artery.

artery A vessel carrying blood away from the heart.

arthralgia Joint pains.

arthritis Inflammation of a joint. This is one of a number of diseases commonly called *rheumatism*. The two most common types of arthritis are *degenerative arthritis*, which is the type seen in older people, accompanied by loss of cartilage about the afflicted joint, stiffness and deformity of the joint, and *rheumatoid arthritis,* which often affects many joints simultaneously and is characterized by pain and limitation of motion.

arthrography X-ray of a joint, after injection of radiopaque material.

arthroplasty The surgical construction or reconstitution of a joint.

arthrorrhagia Hemorrhage into a joint.

articulation The junction of two or more bones.

artificial insemination Insemination by syringe injection directly into the uterus.

artificial respiration The maintenance of breathing by exterior manipulation.

asbestosis A chronic inflammation of the lungs caused by asbestos dust.

ascariasis Infection caused by worms that lodge in the intestine.

Aschoff's bodies Cells seen in the heart muscle of one suffering from heart disease caused by rheumatic fever.

ascites Fluid in the abdomen. It may be caused by a cardiac or kidney condition or by a tumor and is often seen in cirrhosis of the liver.

ascorbic acid Vitamin C.

asepsis A sterile state; free from all germs.

asexual Lack of distinction between male and female.

Asiatic influenza A respiratory virus infection with severe symptoms.

aspermia Absence of sperm in semen.

asphyxia Suffocation.

aspiration Sucking up a fluid, a gas or a solid into a cavity (the lungs, etc.); removal of fluids by suction.

aspirin Acetylsalicylic acid; an analgesic.

astasia The inability to stand in a normal manner because of lack of coordination.

asthenia A lack of vitality characterized by general weakness.

asthma A condition characterized by wheezing, coughing, mucous sputum and difficulty in exhaling air.

astigmatism An eye condition in which vision is distorted because of irregularities in the shape of the cornea or lens of the eye.

astringent Any agent which causes contraction or constriction of tissues.

astroblastoma A malignant brain tumor.

astrocytoma A malignant brain tumor.

asymptomatic Not having symptoms.

Atabrine A substitute for quinine, used in the treatment of malaria.

ataxia Lack of muscle coordination.

atelectasis Incomplete expansion or partial collapse of the lung.

atherosclerosis Hardening of the inner lining of arteries.

athlete's foot A ringworm infection of the feet.

atonia Absence of muscle tone or strength.

atresia Faulty development of an opening in an organ, such as the bile ducts, the rectum, or the vagina.

atrial fibrillation Irregularity of the heart beat, originating in the auricle of the heart.

atrial flutter A very fast heart beat originating from a point in the atrial muscle.

atrium The upper chamber of the heart which receives blood from the veins; the auricle.

atrophy   The withering of an organ or cell.

atropine   A drug which paralyzes nerve endings in the parasympathetic nervous system.

audiometer   An electrical mechanism to measure the sharpness of hearing.

auditory   Referring to the sense of hearing.

aural   Relating to the ear.

auricle   Either of the two upper chambers of the heart which receive blood from the veins. The left auricle admits blood from the lungs and the right auricle from general circulation.

auricular fibrillation   A heart disease in which the upper chambers of the heart are beating very fast and out of time.

auscultation   The detection and study of sounds produced by the lungs, heart, and other organs in order to determine their physical condition.

autoclave   A machine used for sterilizing by a steam process.

autogenous vaccine   A vaccine manufactured from bacteria taken from the body of the individual.

autograft   A graft of tissue from part of an individual's body to another.

avascular   Having a minimum number of blood vessels.

avitaminosis   A disease caused by a lack of vitamins.

axilla   Armpit.

A-Z test   A pregnancy test, utilizing the urine of the pregnant woman (Ascheim-Zondek Test).

bacillary dysentery   An infection of the large bowel caused by germs which enter the body in contaminated food and water.

bacilluria   The presence of bacilli in the urine.

bacillus   A germ shaped like a short rod.

backbone   The spinal column.

bacteremia   Blood poisoning caused by bacteria in the blood stream.

bacteria   Germs.

bactericide   Anything that kills bacteria; an antiseptic.

bacteriogenic   Caused by bacteria.

bacteriologist   A person who specializes in bacteriology.

bacteriology The science and study of bacteria.

bag of waters The liquid surrounding the unborn infant in the womb.

Baker's cyst A cyst in the back of the knee.

balanitis Inflammation of the tip of the penis.

balanus The head of the penis.

band An adhesion.

Banti's disease An enlarged spleen, with anemia, followed by hardening of the liver, jaundice, and an accumulation of fluids in the abdomen.

barbiturates A group of drugs used in calming nerves and inducing sleep.

barbotage The repeated withdrawal and injection of spinal fluid during the administration of spinal anesthesia.

barium An opaque substance which shows up on X-ray films used to show the lining of the intestinal tract during X-rays.

barium enema Injecting a fluid mixture of barium through the rectum before X-raying the large intestine.

Bartholin's glands Small glands in the vagina that pour out a clear mucous secretion to lubricate the vulva during intercourse.

bartholinitis Inflammation of Bartholin's glands frequently caused by gonorrhea.

barylalia Difficult to understand speech in persons with organic brain disease.

basal cell carcinoma A common skin cancer frequently located on the side of the nose or beneath the eyes.

basal metabolism The amount of energy required by the body at rest.

Basedow's disease Overactivity of the thyroid gland.

basiphobia Fear of walking or standing erect.

BCG The abbreviation for an antituberculosis vaccine originally prepared from the Bacillus Calmette-Guérin.

b.d. Twice daily; a term used in prescriptions.

belladonna A medicinal extract of the leaves and root of the "deadly nightshade" plant.

Bell's palsy Paralysis of the muscles of one or both sides of the face.

Benadryl Trademark for an antihistamine medication used to treat allergies.

Benedict's test A chemical test for the presence of sugar in the urine.

benign Not cancerous; not malignant.

Benzedrine A brand name for amphetamine.

benzoin A balsam tree resin which is often administered by steam inhalation for upper respiratory infections.

beriberi A deficiencey disease resulting from lack of vitamin B_1 in the diet.

bicarbonate (HCO_3) A form of carbonic acid present in the blood of all people.

biceps The large muscle on the front of the upper arm.

Bicillin A trademark for benzathine penicillin G, an antibiotic.

bicornuate Having two horns, a common birth defect.

bicuspid A tooth with two cuspids, or points.

b.i.d. Abbreviation for *twice daily*, used in prescriptions.

bidactyly A birth defect characterized by the absence of all fingers or toes except the first and fifth.

bilateral Affecting both sides of the body.

bile A bitter fluid, manufactured in the liver and secreted into the intestines containing chemicals which aid in digestion.

biliousness A digestive disturbance accompanied by headache, nausea, constipation, and other similar complaints.

bilirubin Bile pigment whose presence in the urine usually indicates liver disease.

biliuria Bile in the urine, seen in individuals with jaundice.

bilocular Having two cells or compartments, as in *bilocular* cyst.

biogenesis The theory that living things are produced only from living things.

biokinetics The study of the movement of living organisms.

biologicals Drugs made from living organisms and their by-products.

biopsy The surgical removal of tissue in order to make a diagnosis.

24

biparous Giving birth to twins.

birthmarks Parts of the skin that fail to develop normally before birth.

bisexual 1. Having male and female sex organs; a birth deformity. 2. Being attracted sexually to both males and females.

Black Death Plague.

blackout Loss of consciousness, usually of short duration.

bladder A hollow organ which collects the urine.

blastomycosis A fungus infection producing infection of the skin, bones and other internal organs. Also known as *Gilchrist's disease.*

blepharitis Inflammation of the eyelids.

blepharospasm Spasm of the eyelids producing uncontrolled winking.

blister Collection of fluid under the skin.

blood The red fluid that circulates through the blood vessels. It is composed of red blood cells, white blood cells, blood platelets and plasma.

blood blister A blister that contains blood.

blood coagulation Clotting of the blood.

blood compatibility The ability of one person's blood to mix with another's without causing clots to form.

blood count A test to determine the number of red and white blood cells in the blood.

blood flow The circulation of blood throughout the body.

blood poisoning See **septicemia.**

blood pressure The pressure of the blood against the walls of the vessels of the heart.

blood typing A test to discover a person's blood group.

blue baby A baby born with a structural defect of the heart. The result is a constant recirculation of some of the blood without its being cleansed by the lungs.

B.M.R. Abbreviation for *basal metabolic rate.*

bolus Chewed food ready to be swallowed.

bone marrow The soft material inside long bones.

booster shots An additional vaccination given after the original immunization.

boric acid   A mild antiseptic.

botulism   Severe food poisonings, usually occurring as a result of eating canned foods which have been contaminated by a germ which grows in improperly preserved food.

bowel   The intestine.

bradycardia   An abnormally slow heart rate.

brain   That part of the central nervous system which occupies the inside of the skull.

brain fever   Meningitis or encephalitis.

brain stem   The part of the brain lying between the brain and spinal cord.

brain wave   Electricity generated by the brain.

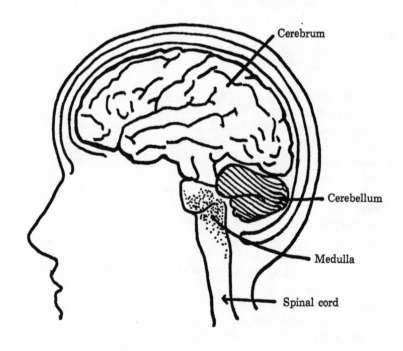

The human brain.

breakbone fever Dengue fever.

breastbone The bone in the front of the chest to which the ribs are attached; also known as the *sternum*.

breech delivery A birth in which the baby is expelled feet first.

Bright's disease Inflammation of the kidneys.

bromhidrosis Body odor.

bromides Drugs used to calm the nerves.

bromism Poisoning with an overdose of bromides. It causes foul breath, dizziness, sleepiness and pimples on the skin.

bronchial asthma Asthma.

bronchial fistula An abnormal connection between a bronchial tube and the chest cavity which surrounds the lung.

bronchial tubes Tubes leading from the nose and mouth to the lungs.

bronchiectasis A coughing sickness, much like chronic bronchitis. Repeated attacks of coughing stretch and dilate the bronchial tubes, often leaving pockets where pus can form.

bronchitis Inflammation of the bronchial tubes.

bronchodilator A medication which enlarges a constricted bronchial tube; often prescribed in acute asthma.

bronchogram X-ray of the bronchial tubes.

bronchopneumonia A form of pneumonia beginning in the bronchial tubes.

bronchoscope An instrument for looking into the bronchial tubes.

brucellosis See **undulant fever.**

Brunschwig's operation Removal of all the sexual organs along with the bladder and rectum, in an attempt to check extensive cancer.

bubo A swollen lymph gland in the groin or armpit.

bubonic plague Plague.

buccal Referring to the inner lining of the cheek.

Buerger's disease An inflammatory disease of the arteries and veins of the legs.

bulbar poliomyelitis Polio affecting the base of the brain.

bunion An enlarged condition of the bone at the ball of the big toe or at some other part of the foot.

burn   The tissue reaction to extreme heat. Classified as: **First degree**: involving only the superficial layers of the skin, as in sunburn. **Second degree**: involving all but the deepest layer of the skin. **Third degree**: involving all layers of the skin and possibly the tissues beneath the skin.

bursa   A small fluid-filled sac which serves as a buffer against friction among joints that touch each other.

bursitis   Inflammation of a bursa.

Butazolidin   A trademark for a medicine used in the treatment of arthritis and bursitis.

buttocks   The two fleshy parts of the body on which one sits.

cachexia   Extreme weight loss resulting from serious disease.

cadaver   A dead body.

caduceus   The insignia of medicine, consisting of a staff with a snake coiled about it.

caffeine   A drug present in coffee, tea, cocoa, chocolate, and some cola drinks which stimulates the heart, nervous system, and kidneys.

caisson disease   Decompression sickness.

caked breasts   Breasts hardened with milk.

calcaneus   The heel bone.

calcification   Deposit of calcium in body tissues, hardening them.

calcium   A chemical found normally in body tissues.

calculus   A stone formed in the body, such as a kidney stone or gall bladder stone.

Caldwell-Luc operation   An operation for the relief of an infected maxillary sinus in the cheek.

calf   The back of the leg.

callus   Thickened skin.

calorie   The heat unit which measures the energy value of food.

calvities   Baldness.

camphor   An oil used in various combinations as a medication.

canal   A channel or duct.

cancer Abnormal growth of cells.

cancerogen A substance which stimulates the formation of cancer.

canine teeth The sharp teeth located just in front of the pre-molars.

canities Gray hair.

canker sore A small ulcer in the mouth or on the lips.

cannonball metastasis Deposits of cancer in the lung, where they produce an X-ray shadow resembling a cannonball.

capillaries Very small blood vessels.

caput medusae Enlarged veins on the abdomen and lower chest, seen in people who have cirrhosis of the liver.

carbarsone A chemical substance used in the treatment of intestinal parasites.

carbohydrate Sugar or starch.

carbolic acid Phenol.

carboluria The presence of phenol in the urine, producing a dark discoloration.

carbuncle A large boil.

carcinogen Any substance which stimulates the formation of cancer.

Carcinoma Cancer.

carcinomatosis Cancer widely spread throughout the body.

cardiac Relating to the heart.

cardiac angina Angina pectoris.

cardiac arrest Stoppage of the heart.

cardiac failure A condition caused by inadequate heart function.

cardiectomy The surgical removal of the upper end of the stomach.

cardiogram A recording of the heart's pulsations.

cardiologist A physician who specializes in diseases of the heart.

cardiomalacia Degeneration of heart muscle.

cardiopulmonary Referring to the heart and lungs.

cardiospasm A muscular spasm of the esophagus and the entrance of the stomach.

cardiovascular Relating to the heart and blood vessels.

carditis Inflammation of the heart.

caries Cavities in the teeth.

carotid artery The principal large artery on each side of the neck.

carpal bones The eight bones of the wrist.

carrier A healthy person who carries germs which can infect and cause disease in another.

cartilage Hard elastic connective tissue covering the ends of bones where they meet to become joints.

cascara sagrada A popular laxative.

casein The principal protein in milk.

castor oil A laxative taken from the seed of the castor bean.

castration Removal of the testicles.

catalepsy A peculiar state of muscular rigidity in which the individual does not move from whatever position he has been placed in.

catamenia Menstruation.

cataract Clouding of the lens of the eye.

catarrh Irritation of a membrane, especially of the respiratory tract, accompanied by secretion of mucus.

catatonia A condition in which the patient will not talk or move and stands or sits in one position and resists attempts to activate motion or speech.

cathartic A medicine to relieve constipation.

catheter A tube used to drain fluid from various cavities of the body.

catheterization The withdrawal of urine from the bladder by a catheter or the insertion of a catheter.

cauda equina The end of the spinal cord composed of the nerves which supply the rectal area.

caudal anesthesia Spinal anesthesia in the region of the sacrum and coccyx used in childbirth and for operations upon the rectum.

caul A term for the sac in which the child lives in the womb during pregnancy.

causalgia A sensation of burning pain, especially in the palms and soles, believed to be due to irritation or disease in the nerves supplying these areas.

caustic Any substance which irritates.

cauterization Destruction of tissue by application of heat or electric current.

cavernitis An inflammation of the shaft of the penis.

cavernous sinus thrombosis An infection and blood clot in the cavernous sinus lying within the skull, behind and above the eyes.

cavity A hole or hollow space.

CDC Abbreviation for *Center for Disease Control.*

cecitis Inflammation of the cecum.

cecostomy An operation to establish a permanent artificial opening into the cecum in order to relieve an intestinal obstruction.

cecum A portion of the bowel on the lower right side of the abdomen.

celiac Relating to the abdomen.

celiac disease A disease of small children associated with intestinal difficulties, malfunction of the pancreas, anemia and inability to grow normally.

cell A mass of protoplasm containing a nucleus.

cellulitis Inflammation of connective tissue, especially the tissues just beneath the skin surface.

cementum The bony cover of the root of teeth.

central nervous system The brain, spinal cord and the nerves.

cephalalgia Headache.

cephalic vein A large vein on the outside of the arm.

cephalopathy Any disease of the head or brain.

cera Wax.

cerebellospinal Referring to the cerebellum and spinal cord.

cerebellum The lower, smaller part of the brain at the base of the skull.

cerebellar speech The slow, slurred, and jerky speech seen in individuals suffering from cerebellar disorders.

cerebral Denotes anything that is related to the cerebrum, the seat of reason in the brain.

cerebral hemorrhage Bleeding in the brain, resulting in stroke or apoplexy.

31

cerebral palsy A neuromuscular disease of the central nervous system.

cerebral paraplegia Paralysis of both legs.

cerebrosclerosis Hardening of brain tissue in the cerebrum.

cerebrospinal fluid Fluid surrounding the brain and spinal cord.

cerebrum The upper part of the brain, controlling conscious thoughts and actions.

cerumen Earwax.

cervical region The neck.

cervicectomy The surgical removal of the cervix.

cervicitis Inflammation of the cervix of the uterus.

cervicovaginitis Inflammation of the cervix of the uterus and the vagina.

cervix The entrance to the womb.

cesarean section Delivery of an infant through an incision in the abdominal wall and the uterus.

chalazion stye.

chancre A small, hard, painless sore. The first visible symptom of syphilis.

chancroid A venereal disease in which the chancre is soft.

change of life Menopause.

cheilitis Inflammation of the lips.

chemotherapy Prevention or treatment of disease through chemicals.

chest That part of the body extending from the base of the neck down to the diaphragm.

chicken pox Varicella; a common childhood disease caused by a specific virus.

chilblains An inflammation of the skin and the tissues under the skin caused by cold.

chill A sensation of cold, accompanied by shivering.

Chinese restaurant syndrome Sensation of burning pressure about the face and chest, often accompanied by headache, produced by the eating of monosodium L-glutamate (used in Chinese cooking) on an empty stomach.

chiropodist Foot specialist, who treats minor ailments of the feet.

chloral hydrate A powerful sleep-producing drug.

chlorhydria Excess stomach acidity.

chloroform A drug which produces anesthesia when inhaled.

Chloromycetin Trademark for chloramphenicol, a powerful antibiotic.

chlorophyll The green coloring substance in plants.

chlorpromazine (Thorazine) A tranquilizing medication used to combat nausea and vomiting. It is also used to calm the nerves.

choked disk Swelling of the retina at the site where the nerve enters.

cholecyst The gall bladder.

cholecystectomy The surgical removal of the gall bladder.

cholecystitis Inflammation of the gall bladder.

cholecystography X-ray of the gall bladder after it has been made visual by the administration of a dye, either by mouth or by injection.

cholecystojejunostomy An operation to unite the gall bladder and the jejunum (small intestine).

cholecystostomy The establishment of an opening into the gall bladder, in order to drain it.

cholecystotomy Incision into the gall bladder to remove gallstones.

choledochitis Inflammation of the bile duct.

choledocholithotomy The surgical removal of stones from the bile duct.

cholera An infection which chiefly involves the small intestine. The main symptoms are severe, constantly flowing diarrhea, vomiting, cramps in the muscles, and suppression of the flow of urine from the kidneys.

cholesterol A fatty substance found in all animal fats and oils.

cholografin An opaque dye, which, when injected into a vein, will show the interior outline of the gall bladder and bile ducts on X-rays.

choluria Bile in urine.

chondral Pertaining to cartilage.

chondritis The inflammation of a cartilage.

chondroma A benign tumor of cartilage.

chondrosarcoma A malignant tumor of cartilage.

chorditis The inflammation of a cord—the vocal cord, or the spermatic cord which connects with the testicle.

chordotomy An operation to relieve pain, performed upon the spinal cord.

chorea St. Vitus' dance. A disease of the nervous system which causes involuntary twitching of various parts of the body.

chorioadenoma A tumor within the uterus.

choriocarcinoma A highly malignant tumor found most commonly in the uterus and testis.

chorion A membrane surrounding the unborn child in the womb.

chorioretinitis An inflammation in the back of the eye.

chorioretinopathy Disease of the eye involving both the choroid and retina.

choroid A membrane of the eyeball containing blood vessels.

choroiditis Inflammation of the choroid.

Christmas disease A hereditary disease having many of the characteristics of hemophilia.

chromatopathy Any abnormality of the color of the skin.

chromatosis Abnormal pigmentation in the tissues.

chromosome The body within a cell which controls heredity.

chronic Persistent, repeated; the opposite of acute.

chrysarobin A powder medication for the treatment of psoriasis, and certain fungal infections of the skin.

chrysotherapy Treatment with gold compounds.

chyle A milky-white, partially digested fat which is transported from the intestines through lymph vessels.

chylothorax Chyle in the chest cavity.

chyluria The presence of chyle or lymph in the urine.

cicatrix Scar tissue.

cilia Eyelashes.

cincophen A chemical sometimes used in the treatment of gout and rheumatism.

cinerea Gray matter of the brain or spinal cord.

cineroentgenography Motion picture X-rays.

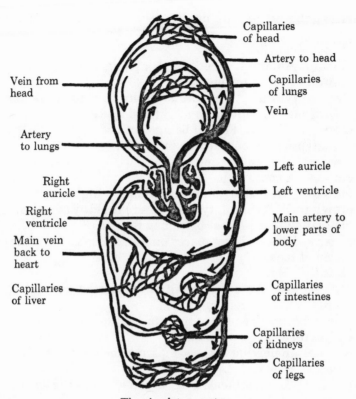

The circulatory system.

circinate   Circular or ringlike.

circle of Willis   A group of arteries surrounding the base of the brain.

circulation   The passage of blood from the heart to all parts of the body and its return from the tissues to the heart.

circulation time   The rate of blood flow.

circumcision   The surgical removal of the foreskin, which covers the head of the penis.

cirrhosis   Hardening of an organ as the result of inflammation or other disease occuring most often in the kidney and liver.

citric acid   The acid found in citrus fruits, such as orange, lemon, and grapefruit.

citronella oil An oil used to repel mosquitoes and other insects.

clap Gonorrhea.

clasmocytoma See **reticulum cell sarcoma.**

claudication Lameness.

claustrophilia An abnormal desire to shut doors and windows and be shut up in a confined space.

claustrophobia Fear of being confined

claustrum An obstruction or barrier.

clavicle The collarbone.

clavus A corn.

clawfoot A foot with an exceptionally high arch.

clawhand A deformity of the hand caused by nerve paralysis.

clearance test A test of kidney function.

cleavage lines Lines placed on the skin to indicate the direction of tension.

cleft lip Harelip.

cleft palate A birth deformity in which the roof of the mouth fails to join its midline.

cleptomania See **kleptomania.**

climacteric The menopause.

clinical Referring to the symptoms and course of a disease as observed by the physician.

clitoris The erect female sex organ which is the female counterpart of the penis.

clitoritis Inflammation of the clitoris.

clonic Referring to jerky muscle contractions or spasms.

closed-chest massage A technique used to revive a heart which has stopped beating.

closed reduction The setting of a broken bone, performed without making a surgical incision.

closure The suturing of a wound.

clot The mass that forms when blood clots.

clubfoot A deformity of the foot in which the heel or the ball of the foot, or one edge of it, does not touch the ground.

coagulation The formation of a clot, as in blood.

coalescence The union of two or more parts or things previously separate.

coal miner's disease Anthracosilicosis; a lung inflammation caused by inhaling coal dust.

coaptation The proper union of displaced parts in a wound.

cobalt A metal element used in the treatment of cancer.

cocaine A narcotic drug used as a local anesthetic.

coccidioidomycosis A bump caused by inhaling certain spores of a fungus. It is also known as desert fever, San Joaquin fever, valley fever, or the bumps.

coccidioidosis Coccidioidomycosis.

coccus A round-shaped germ.

coccygectomy The surgical excision of the coccyx.

coccyx Tail bone.

cochlea A part of the inner ear which houses the main organ of hearing.

codeine A pain relieving drug, derived from opium.

cod-liver oil An oil obtained from the livers of cod and halibut very rich in vitamins A and D.

coitus Sexual intercourse.

coitus interruptus Sexual intercourse in which the penis is withdrawn just before ejaculation.

colchicine A drug used in the treatment of gout.

cold sore A sore of the lips caused by a mild virus infection.

colectomy The excision of a part of or all of the large bowel.

colic A severe abdominal pain.

colic, renal Severe, often excruciating, sudden pain in the kidney region and along the ureter, caused by a kidney stone.

colitis Inflammation of the large bowel.

collagen diseases Diseases involving the connective tissues of the body.

collarbone The clavicle.

Colles' fracture A frequently encountered fracture of the wrist, involving the radius bone.

colloid gold test A test for syphilis of the nervous system.

collum Neck.

coloboma Any deformity of the eye.

colon The large bowel or intestine, extending from the cecum to the anus.

coloproctostomy An operation to form a new passage between the colon and the rectum.

Colorado tick fever A virus infection transmitted by the bite of an infected tick.

color blindness Inability to distinguish one or more colors.

colostomy A surgical operation in which the large bowel is brought out to form a permanent opening (an artificial anus) in the wall of the abdomen.

colostomy bag A rubber bag worn as a belt, especially constructed to receive the bowel movements from a colostomy opening.

colostrum The milky fluid that flows from the breasts a few days before or after childbirth. It is different from regular breast milk.

colotomy A surgical incision into the colon.

colpectomy The surgical removal of the vagina.

colpitis Inflammation of the vagina.

colpocele A hernia in the vagina.

colpoplasty The surgical repair of a tear in the wall of the vagina, a condition common following difficult childbirth.

colporrhaphy Colpoplasty.

colposcopy Examination of the vagina with an instrument called the *speculum.*

coma Unconsciousness from which the patient cannot be aroused.

comatose Being unconscious.

comedo Blackhead.

comedocarcinoma A type of breast cancer in which the malignant cells are in the breast ducts.

comminuted fracture One in which the bone is shattered into several pieces.

commissurotomy An operation in which a deformed heart valve is cut to permit a normal flow of blood.

communicable diseases Diseases which are transmissible from one person to another.

Compazine Trademark for a drug used to control nausea and vomiting.

compound fracture A fracture in which the skin covering the bone is broken.

conceive To become pregnant.

conception Pregnancy.

concha The hollow portion of the external ear.

concussion of the brain A bruise of the brain the result of a blow or fall.

condom A sheath of thin rubber worn over the penis during sexual intercourse to prevent infection or pregnancy.

condyloma A wartlike growth near the external sex organs or the anus.

congelation Frost-bite.

congenital defects Birth deformities.

congestion An excessive accumulation of blood in any part of the body or excess phlegm in the lungs.

congestive heart failure A state in which congestion exists in blood vessels as a result of heart failure.

conization The surgical removal of the *conjunctiva*, the membrane covering the globe and lids of the eye.

conjunctivitis Inflammation of the *conjunctiva*, the membrane covering the globe and lids of the eye.

consolidation The process of becoming firm or solid, as a lung in pneumonia. A *consolidated lung* is one in which the air cells are filled with fluid, mucus or pus.

constipation Difficult bowel movement.

constriction Narrowing.

consultant A physician, usually a specialist, called in to see a patient by another physician.

consultation A deliberation between two or more physicians concerning the treatment of a patient.

consumption Tuberculosis of the lungs.

contact dermatitis A skin disorder resulting from contact with some outside substance such as poison ivy.

contact ulcer A superficial ulcer on one or both sides of the larynx.

continence Self-restraint in regard to sexual intercourse or bladder or bowel function.

contraception The prevention of conception during sexual intercourse.

contracture The shortening of a muscle, tendon or other

structure so that it cannot be readily straightened.

contusion   A bruise.

convalescence   The recovery period after an illness or operation.

convolution   A fold of any organ, especially of the folds of brain tissue in the cerebrum.

convulsion   A violent attack of uncontrollable muscle spasms caused by a brain irritation.

convulsive disorders   Any disease associated with recurring convulsions.

copulation   Sexual intercourse.

cordectomy   The surgical removal of any cord such as the vocal fold.

corium   The lower layer of the skin.

corn   A thickening of the skin on the toes.

cornea   The transparent membrane in the front of the eyeball.

corneal transplant   An operation in which a section of the cornea is substituted for one already existing.

cornu   A crescent-shaped organ near the entrance of the fallopian tubes.

cornual pregnancy   Pregnancy occurring in the cornu of the uterus.

coronary   A heart attack.

coronary arteries   Arteries that supply the heart muscle.

coronary occlusion   A blockage that stops the flow of blood through the coronary arteries; a form of heart attack.

coronary thrombosis   A heart attack, caused by a blood clot in the coronary arteries.

corpus cavernosum penis   The spongy tissue forming the shaft of the penis.

corpuscle   Blood cell.

Corrigan's pulse   A pounding pulse found in people who have a diseased aortic valve in the heart.

cortex   The surface layer of an organ such as the kidney or adrenal gland.

cortex renis   The cortex of a kidney.

cortin   The hormone of the cortex of the adrenal gland.

cortisone A hormone produced by the cortex of the adrenal gland.

coryza Inflammation of the mucous membranes of the nose.

costal cartilage The cartilage which connects the ribs to the breastbone.

costalgia Pain in the ribs.

costectomy The excision of a rib or a part of one.

costive Pertaining to constipation.

cough syncope Fainting following a severe attack of coughing.

Coumadin Trademark for *warfarin*, an anticoagulant medication used by those who have had a coronary thrombosis, and to thin the blood of those who show a tendency toward blood clots and phlebitis.

counterirritant An agent that produces inflammation of the skin in order to counteract a deeper inflammation.

coupling A heart irregularity in which each normal heart beat is followed by a premature contraction.

Cowper's glands The glands located at the entrance of the bladder.

cowpox The viral disease of cattle which, when transmitted to man by vaccination, gives immunity against smallpox.

cox The hip.

coxalgia Pain in hip joint.

coxa valga A deformity of the thighbone in the hip region in which the angle between the neck and the shaft is increased.

coxa vara A deformity of the thighbone in the hip region in which the neck of the thighbone is bent downward.

Coxsackie disease A disease which gives the appearance of infantile paralysis or meningitis but clears up in a few days.

cramps A sudden, involuntary, painful contraction of a muscle.

cranial Pertaining to the skull.

cranial nerves The twelve nerves originating from the brain.

craniopathy Any disease of the head.

craniopharyngioma A tumor at the base of the brain near the pituitary gland.

cranioplasty A surgical correction of defects in the cranial bones.

craniosynostosis Premature hardening of the skull present at or shortly after birth.

craniotabes A degeneration of bones of the skull, often found in infants having rickets and other diseases.

craniotomy Any operation performed upon the skull.

cranium The skull.

creeping pneumonia Migratory pneumonia.

creeping ulcer An ulcer with a wavy, snake-like border.

cremaster The muscle which supports the testicles.

cretinism A condition originating before birth or in early infancy in which mental and physical development are stunted due to a severe thyroid deficiency.

cribriform Perforated like a sieve.

cricothyroid The muscle which causes the vocal cords to constrict.

crocodile tears syndrome A profuse flow of tears seen in certain individuals with facial paralysis, when they taste strongly flavored food.

cross-eye The result of imbalance of the muscles which control eyeball movement.

cross matching of blood The technique used to determine whether or not the blood to be given to a patient will mix safely with his own blood without clotting.

croton oil An extremely powerful laxative.

croup An inflammation of the larynx accompanied by hoarse coughing, and labored breathing.

crown (of a tooth) The part of the tooth covered with enamel.

crus A leg.

crust Scab.

cryanesthesia Loss of sensation of cold by the skin.

cryesthesia Extreme sensitivity to cold.

cryogenics The science of cold and its uses in treating illness.

cryosurgery Surgery performed by freezing diseased tissues.

cryotherapy The use of cold in the treatment of disease.

cryptorchidectomy Removal of an undescended testicle.

cryptorchidism Failure of one or both testicles to descend normally into the scrotum.

crystalline lens The lens of the eye.

crystalluria The presence of crystals in the urine.

CSF Abbreviation for *cerebrospinal fluid*.

cubitus The forearm.

cuboid An ankle bone.

culdoscope An instrument inserted through the vagina into the abdominal cavity to examine the internal organs.

culture Germs artifically grown.

curet A spoon-shaped instrument used for scraping away tissues.

curettage The scraping out of the contents of a cavity, such as the uterus.

cursive epilepsy A form of epilepsy characterized by running to oblivious obstacles.

curvature of the spine A general term applied to many abnormal spine conditions such as scoliosis, kyphosis, and lordosis.

Cushing's disease A kind of brain tumor.

cusp 1. The pointed part of a tooth. 2. A leaf of a heart valve.

cuspid A canine tooth.

cutaneous Relating to the skin.

cutis The skin.

cyanosis A bluish appearance of the skin, indicating a lack of oxygen in the blood.

cyclodialysis An operation to relieve the pressure within the eyeball in glaucoma.

cyclopropane An anesthetic gas.

cyclotomy An operation for the relief of glaucoma.

cyesis Pregnancy.

cynophobia An abnormal fear of dogs.

cyst A sac enclosing a fluid.

cystadenocarcinoma A type of cancer containing many cysts.

cystalgia Pain in the urinary bladder.

cystectomy Removal of a cyst or of the urinary bladder.

cystic fibrosis A childhood disease characterized by the failure of the glands that secrete mucus and digestive juices.

cystitis Inflammation of the urinary bladder.

cystocele A hernia of the bladder causing it to protrude into the vagina.

cystogram An X-ray of the urinary bladder.

cystoid Cyst-like.

cystolithiasis Stones in the urinary bladder.

cystolithotomy The surgical removal of a urinary bladder stone.

cystoprostatectomy The excision of the urinary bladder and the prostate.

cystosarcoma phylloides A benign tumor of the breast.

cystoscope An instrument for examining the inside of the bladder.

cystotomy 1. An incision into the urinary bladder or gallbladder. 2. An incision into the lens of the eye for the extraction of a cataract.

dacnomania An impulse to kill.

dacryocystitis Inflammation of the tear sac of the eye.

dacryocystectomy The removal of any part of the tear sac.

dactylomegaly A condition in which one or more of the fingers or toes is abnormally large.

D and C Dilatation of the cervix and curettage of the lining of the uterus performed in order to diagnose cancer of the uterus.

dandruff Small scales of skin on the scalp.

Darvon Trademark for a non-habit-forming, pain-relieving drug.

D.C. Doctor of Chiropractic.

D.D.S. Doctor of Dental Surgery.

debridement Removal of dead tissue.

44

decalcification The process of losing calcium from the bones or teeth.

decapsulization The surgical removal of an enveloping membrane of an organ.

dechloridation Removal of salt from the diet.

deciduous teeth The baby teeth.

decompensation Heart failure.

decompression sickness A condition caused by the formation of nitrogen bubbles in the blood due to an abrupt reduction in atmospheric pressure.

decrudescence The subsiding of a disease.

decubitus ulcer Bedsore.

defecation The elimination of waste from the bowel.

defibrillation A maneuver to stop irregular beating of the heart.

deficiency disease A disease caused by a lack of vitamins or minerals in the body.

defloration The loss of virginity.

degeneration Deterioration of tissues.

deglutition Swallowing.

dehiscence Splitting open.

dehydration The condition that results when an excessive or abnormal amount of water is removed from the body.

delirium A mental disturbance in which the sufferer is confused and disturbed by hallucinations.

delirium tremens A delirious condition brought on by alcohol poisoning characterized by hallucinations and trembling.

deltoid The triangular muscle that covers the shoulder and stretches down the upper part of the arm.

dementia Mental deterioration.

Demerol Trademark for a synthetic pain killer.

demulcent A soothing, medicated ointment.

denervate To remove a nerve.

dengue fever A virus disease characterized by severe pain in muscles, joints, and bones, and by high fever.

dens A tooth.

dentalgia Toothache.

dentigerous cyst   A cyst, in the jaw bones, coming from a developing tooth.

dentine   The chalky part of the tooth found under the enamel and cement of the root.

dentition   Teething.

depilate   To remove hair.

depilatory   Any preparation used to remove hair from the body.

depressant   A medicine which diminishes activity.

Dercum's disease   A disease associated with painful areas in the fatty tissue beneath the skin.

derma   Skin.

dermabrasion   The removal of skin by mechanical means.

dermatitis   An inflammation of the skin.

dermatologist   A skin specialist.

dermatoneurosis   A skin rash caused by emotional upset.

dermatophytosis   Athlete's foot.

dermis   The lower layer of the skin.

desmitis   Inflammation of a ligament.

detachment of the retina   Separation of the retina from the choroid.

devascularize   To cut off the blood supply to an organ.

deviated septum   A defect in the wall separating the two portions of the nose.

Dexedrine   Amphetamine.

dextrose   A form of sugar found in the blood.

diabetes   A disease caused by insufficient production of insulin by the pancreas.

diaphragm   A wide muscle which separates the abdominal and chest cavities of the body.

diarrhea   Loose bowels.

diastole   The resting of the heart between beats.

diathermy   The use of high-frequency electric current to apply heat to deep seated tissues of the body.

Dick test   A test to discover susceptibility to scarlet fever.

dietetics   The science of regulating diet in order to preserve health.

Dietl's crisis   Excruciating pain in the kidney region, brought on by a twist of a ureter.

digestant An agent which promotes digestion.

digestion The process by which food is converted into soluble form for absorption into the tissues and cells of the body.

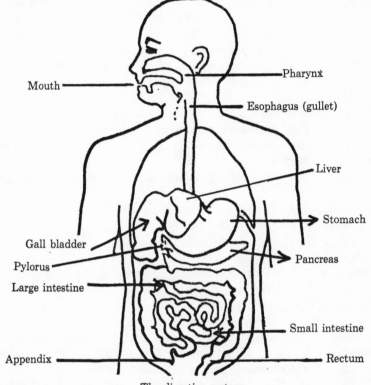

The digestive system.

digit A finger or toe.

digitalis A drug used in treating heart failure and dropsy.

Dilantin A trademark for *diphenylhydantoin*, an anticonvulsant drug used in the treatment of epilepsy.

dilation The expansion of an organ, such as the cervix, with an instrument to aid in further examination.

diphtheria An infectious disease characterized by sore throat and interference with breathing.

47

diplegia Paralysis of two arms or two legs

diplopia Seeing double.

dipsomania Insatiable thirst for alcoholic beverages.

disarticulation Amputation of a limb through the joint.

disease, congenital A disease that is present at birth.

disease, degenerative One in which some part of the body wears out.

disease, psychosomatic Any disease in which the emotions bring on the symptoms.

disk A layer of cartilage between the vertebrae.

dislocation The displacement of one or more bones from a joint.

disseminated sclerosis Multiple sclerosis.

diuresis The excessive excretion of urine.

diuretic An agent that increases the quantity of urine.

diurnal Occurring in the daytime.

diverticulitis An inflammation of a diverticulum of the bowel.

diverticulum A small pouch which sometimes develops on the smooth wall of the bowel.

D.M.D. Doctor of Dental Medicine.

dolor Pain.

doraphobia A fear of touching the skin or fur of animals.

dorsal Pertaining to the back.

dosage The proper amount of a medicine or other agent for a given patient or condition.

double pneumonia Pneumonia involving both lungs.

douche Refers to the cleansing of the vagina with a solution of some chemical in warm water.

Dramamine The trade name for dimenhydrinate, a drug used in the prevention and treatment of motion sickness.

Drinker respirator An iron lung.

dropsy Abnormal accumulation of water in tissues and cavities.

drug fever Fever resulting from the administration of a drug.

dry labor Early rupture of the membranes during childbirth.

DTs Delirium tremens.

duct A tube or canal through which something flows.

duodenal ulcer Ulcer of the duodenum.

duodenitis Inflammation of the duodenum.

duodenum The first portion of the small intestine.

Dupuytren's contracture A painless, chronic contracting of the hand, marked by thickening of the tissue beneath the skin of the palm of the hand and an inability to fully extend the fingers.

dura mater The outer covering of the brain.

D.V.M. Doctor of Veterinary Medicine.

dysaphea Disordered sense of touch.

dysentery Inflammation of the colon.

dysfunction Abnormal function of an organ.

dyslalia Impaired power of speech.

dysmenorrhea Pain at the time of menstruation.

dyspareunia Painful sexual intercourse.

dyspepsia Indigestion.

dysphagia Impaired swallowing.

dyspnea Difficult labored breathing.

dysstasia Difficulty in standing.

dystrophy Degeneration.

dysuria Painful urination.

Eagle test A test for syphilis.

ear The organ of hearing, composed of the external ear, the middle ear, and the inner ear.

eardrum The tympanic membrane which separates the external ear from the middle ear.

ecchymosis A bruise.

ECG Abbreviation for *electrocardiogram*.

echinococcus cyst A cyst (usually in the liver) caused by infestation with a worm.

eclampsia A serious convulsive condition occurring in pregnant women.

ecthyma A skin disease characterized by large, flat pus cells that ulcerate.

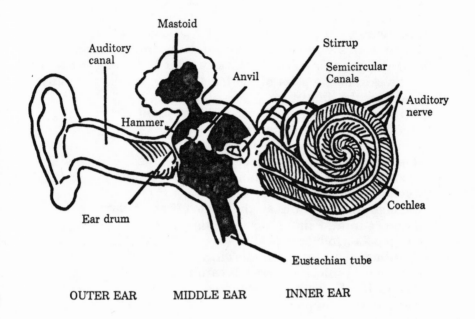

Mastoid

Auditory
canal

Anvil

Stirrup

Semicircular
Canals

Auditory
nerve

Hammer

Cochlea

Ear drum

Eustachian tube

OUTER EAR   MIDDLE EAR   INNER EAR

The ear.

ectopic Out of place.

ectopic pregnancy A pregnancy in which the fetus develops outside of the womb such as in the fallopian tube.

eczema A skin disease or disorder whose cause or origin is unknown.

edema Abnormal amounts of fluid in body tissues causing swelling.

edentulous Without teeth.

EEG See *electroencephalography*.

EENT An abbreviation which means "eye, ear, nose, and throat" and is used to indicate a doctor or clinic which specializes in disorders of these organs.

efferent nerves Nerves which originate in the central nervous system and go out toward the organs.

ejaculation An emission, such as takes place in the male during orgasm.

EKG An abbreviation for *electrocardiogram*.

electrocardiogram A tracing produced by the *electrocardiograph*, a device which records the electrical current created by the beating of the heart.

electrocardiography Recording and interpreting the electrical activity of the heart.

electrocautery The burning of tissue with electric current.

electroencephalography Recording brain waves.

electrolysis Hair removal by the use of an electric needle.

electromyograph An instrument which records the electrical impulses that pass through a muscle as it contracts and relaxes.

electroshock therapy The use of electric current to treat certain mental illnesses.

electrosurgery The use of an electric current during surgery.

elephantiasis Huge swelling of the legs, scrotum, and occasionally other parts of the body, due to an obstruction of the lymph channels.

elixir A pleasant-tasting solution, used to disguise the taste of bitter medicines.

emaciation Extreme thinness.

embolectomy The surgical removal of an embolus.

embolism Obstruction of a blood vessel by a blood clot or by any foreign body floating loose in the bloodstream.

embolus Anything carried along in the blood stream that causes the sudden blocking of a vein or artery.

embryo The developing child in its mother's womb, from the time of conception to about the third month of pregnancy. Thereafter, until birth, it is called a fetus.

emesis Vomiting.

emetic A substance used to induce vomiting.

emmenagogue A drug used to bring on menstruation.

emollient Any substance that soothes or softens the skin or internal membranes.

emphysema The condition which exists when the normal air spaces in the lungs are enlarged.

empyema A collection of pus in a cavity or organ.

encanthis A tumor in the corner of the eye.

encephalalgia Headache.

encephalogram An X-ray picture of the brain.

encephalomyelitis Inflammation of the brain and spinal cord.

encephalon The brain.

encysted Enclosed in a cyst or capsule.

endarteritis An inflammation of the inner lining of an artery.

endocarditis Inflammation of the valves and lining of the heart.

endocardium The membrane lining the chambers of the heart.

endocrine glands Any of the ductless glands, such as the adrenals, the thyroid, or the pituitary, which secrete directly into the bloodstream.

endometritis Inflammation of the inner lining of the womb.

endometrium The mucous membrane lining the inner surface of the uterus.

endoscope An instrument used for the visual examination of the interior of a body cavity.

endothelioma Any tumor originating from cells which line blood vessels, lymph channels, and various body cavities.

endothermy Diathermy.

endotracheal anesthesia General anesthesia administered by a tube which conducts gas directly into the windpipe.

enema An injection of liquid into the lower bowel through the rectum.

enervation Weakness.

enterectomy The surgical removal of part of the intestine.

enteric Relating to the intestines.

enteric fever Typhoid fever.

enteritis Any acute or chronic inflammation of the intestines.

enteroenterostomy An operation in which an opening is made to join two parts of the intestine.

52

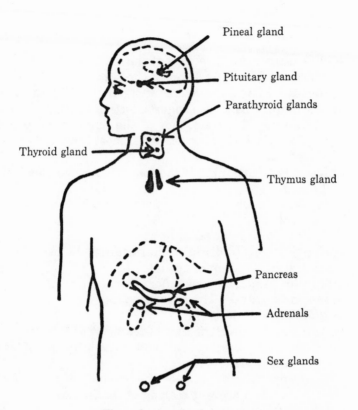

The endocrine glands.

entoptic Referring to the internal parts of the eye.

entropion A condition in which the eyelashes rub against the eyeball.

enuresis Bedwetting.

enzyme A substance promoting a chemical change.

enzymolysis A chemical change produced by an enzyme.

eonism Transvestitism.

ependyma The innermost lining of the brain and spinal cord cavities.

ependymoma A type of tumor of the central nervous system.

ephedrine A drug with action similar to adrenalin often used to counteract shock and stimulate the heart muscle.

epicardia The part of the esophagus between the diaphragm and the stomach.

epicranium   The coverings of the skull.

epidermis   The outer layer of the skin.

epidermoid carcinoma   A cancer originating in the skin.

epidermophytosis   A fungus infection of the skin.

epididymitis   Inflammation of the epididymis (a group of tubules attached to the testicles) most frequently caused by gonorrhea.

epigastric   Pertaining to the space in the abdomen just below the ribs.

epiglottis   A piece of elastic cartilage which forms the lid of the voice box.

epilation   The removal of hair.

epilepsy   A brain disorder characterized by periodic convulsions and loss of consciousness.

epileptic   A person who suffers from epilepsy.

epinephric gland   The adrenal gland.

epinephrine   Adrenalin.

epiphora   A persistent flow of tears.

epiploectomy   Surgical removal of the large pad of fat which covers the intestines.

episiotomy   The slitting of the vaginal walls to facilitate childbirth and prevent tearing of the tissues.

epistaxis   Nosebleed.

epithelioma   Any benign tumor of the skin.

epizoic   Relating to parasites which live on the skin.

eponychium   The cuticle of the nails.

epsom salt   Magnesium sulfate; used as a laxative or as a wet dressing.

epulis   Any benign tumor beneath the gums.

Equanil   A trademark for meprobamate, a tranquilizer drug.

Erb's palsy   Paralysis of the nerves supplying the arm resulting from an injury during childbirth.

erection   Enlargement and rigidification of the penis.

ergot   A fungus that grows on grains and cereals and is used to aid the uterus to contract after childbirth.

ergotamine   A derivative of ergot, helpful in relieving migraine headaches.

ergotism   Ergot poisoning, the result of an overdose of ergot.

eructation Belching.

erugation The removal of wrinkles.

erugatory A substance that removes wrinkles.

eruption A skin rash.

erysipelas A skin disease caused by streptococcal infection. The skin looks fiery red, glazed, and swollen.

erythema A redness of the skin occurring in patches caused by heat, certain drugs, and infections.

erythroblastosis fetalis An anemia of the newborn, who sometimes appear so jaundiced they are called "yellow babies." The cause is the Rh factor.

erythrocyte A red blood cell.

esophagectomy The surgical removal of the esophagus.

esophagitis Inflammation of the esophagus.

esophagogastrostomy An operation in which a new connection is made between the esophagus and the stomach.

esophagogram An X-ray of the esophagus.

esophagoscopy The examination of the esophagus with a specially designed instrument inserted in the mouth.

esophagus The food pipe, or gullet.

ESP Extrasensory perception.

essential hypertension A disease in which blood pressure is above normal.

EST Abbreviation for *electroshock therapy*.

estrogen The female sex hormone, manufactured by the ovaries.

ether A thin, colorless liquid used as an anesthetic.

ethisterone A hormone medication given in certain cases to prevent miscarriage.

ethmoid A bone at the base and front of the skull which forms the upper part of the nose.

ethmoiditis Sinusitis.

ethylene A gas used as an anesthetic.

eunuch A male whose testes or testes and penis have been removed.

eustachian tube The tube leading from the back of the throat to the ear.

euthanasia The killing of a patient with a hopeless disease; mercy-killing.

evacuate To empty, such as the pus from an abscess.

evagination The bulging out of tissue.

eventration The bulging of intestines through a rupture in the wall of the abdomen.

Ewing's tumor A type of bone cancer, which attacks the long bones of the body.

excavation Cutting a hole in an organ.

exchange transfusion The replacement of most or all of the recipient's blood in small amounts.

excise To cut out surgically.

excitant Any drug which stimulates the activity of an organ.

excrement Feces; stool.

excretion The discharge from the body of waste products, including feces, sweat, and urine.

exitus Death.

exodontia The art of extracting teeth.

exogenous Arising from a source outside the body; opposite of endogenous.

exophthalmos Popeyes; usually the result of goiter.

exostosis A bony outgrowth from the surface of a bone.

exotoxin The poison excreted by living germs.

exotorphia A form of crossed eyes in which one eye turns outward.

expectorant A medication that helps a patient bring up and spit out excessive phlegm.

expiration Breathing out.

explantation The removal of living tissue for examination.

exploratory operation An operation performed for the purpose of diagnosis.

exsanguination The loss of huge quantities of blood.

extension Traction of a fractured or dislocated limb.

extensor A muscle which extends or stretches a limb or part; opposite of flexor.

external os The portion of the cervix of the uterus that opens into the vaginal canal.

extirpation The surgical removal of all or part of an organ.

extramural Outside the wall of an organ.

extrasystole An extra heartbeat.

extrauterine pregnancy A pregnancy which takes place outside the uterus.

extravasation A condition in which body fluid leaves its normal channel.

extremity A limb.

extrinsic Originating outside.

extrinsic asthma Asthma caused by a foreign body.

extrophy Deformity of an organ.

eye The organ of sight.

eye teeth The sharp canine teeth in the upper jaw.

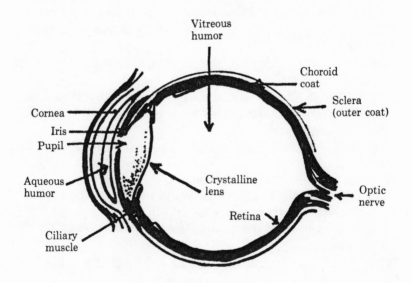

The human eye.

F.A.C.D.   Fellow of the American College of Dentists.

face   The front part of the head, including the forehead and jaws, but not the ears.

face presentation   A position during labor in which the face of the unborn child appears at the vagina.

facial nerve   The seventh cranial nerve, supplying the muscles, surfaces and organs of the face.

facial palsy   The partial or total weakness of the muscles of the face.

F.A.C.P.   Fellow of the American College of Physicians.

F.A.C.S.   Fellow of the American College of Surgeons.

fainting   A temporary suspension of consciousness.

falling sickness   Epilepsy.

fallopian tubes   The two tubes from the ovaries to the uterus.

false hernia   A hernia that has no sac covering its contents.

false labor   Uterine contractions coming several days before real labor.

familial disease   Any disease occurring in several members of the same family.

fascia   Tough, fibrous tissue located in various places throughout the body and serving as a covering for many muscles and internal organs.

fascia lata   The deep sheet of tissue covering the big muscles of the thigh.

fascitis   Inflammation of the fascia.

fatty degeneration   Degeneration of an organ and replacement of its normal contents by fat.

fauces   The back of the mouth; the passage between mouth and throat.

favus   A ringworm infection of the skin, usually the scalp.

febrile   Feverish.

feces   The excrement from the bowels.

fecundity   Fertility.

fellatio   Sexual stimulation of the penis with the mouth.

felon   An abscess of the fingertip.

femoral   Pertaining to the thighbone or the thigh.

femoral artery   The main artery supplying the thigh and leg.

femoral hernia   A hernia located just beneath the crease of the groin.

femur   The thighbone.

fenestration   An operation to relieve deafness.

ferric   Pertaining to, or containing, iron.

ferrotherapy   Treatment of disease with iron and iron compounds.

fertility   The ability to bear children.

fester   To form an abscess containing pus.

fetal   Pertaining to the unborn child.

fetation   Pregnancy.

fetus   The unborn child during the later part of pregnancy.

fever   A body temperature above 98.6° F.

fever blister   A mild virus infection requiring no treatment.

fiber   Any threadlike structure.

fibrillation   Tremor of a muscle commonly applied to the heart muscle and connoting an irregular heart action.

fibroadenoma   A type of benign tumor frequently encountered in the breast.

fibroid tumor   A common benign tumor of the uterus.

fibroma   A benign tumor composed mainly of fibrous tissue.

fibrositis   Inflammation of fibrous or connective tissue of the muscles anywhere in the body outside of the joints.

fibrous   Containing fibers.

fibula   The outer leg bone.

filiform   Thread-shaped.

fissure   A split between adjoining parts of an organ.

fissured tongue   A condition in which there are deep furrows in the mucous membrane of the tongue.

fistula   A passageway between body parts that should not be there.

fistulectomy   The surgical removal of a fistula.

fistulization   The formation of a fistula.

fixation   The immobilization of a part of the body, such as a dislocated bone.

flap   A partially detached portion of skin or other tissue.

flat foot   An arch of the foot which is not properly curved.

flatulence   An excess of air or gas in the stomach or intestines.

59

flatus Gas or air in the stomach or intestines which can be expelled through the mouth or anus.

flexion The bending of a joint.

flexor Any muscle that bends a part of the body.

floating kidney A kidney that moves from its natural position.

flu Short for influenza.

fluoridation The adding of fluorine to drinking water in an attempt to cut down on tooth cavities.

fluoroscope A type of X-ray machine in which the interior of the body shows up on a screen.

fluoroscopy The examination of internal body structures with a fluoroscope.

flutter A heart condition in which the heart beats at a rate of 200 to 400 times a minute.

fold A doubling of a membrane or other part of the body.

Foley catheter A tube used in the urinary bladder.

folic acid A chemical constituent of the body used in treating certain types of anemia.

follicle A small sac or gland which secretes.

folliculitis Inflammation of a follicle.

fontanelles The two soft spots in the infant's skull.

food poisoning Poisoning due to contaminated food.

foot-and-mouth disease A contagious disease of animals which is sometimes transmitted to humans.

foot drop A falling foot caused by paralysis of the muscles which flex the foot or a cut tendon.

foramen A perforation or opening, especially in a bone.

forefinger The index finger.

forensic medicine Legal medicine.

foreskin The skin over the head of the penis.

formaldehyde A strong disinfectant used to fumigate as well as preserve.

formication An abnormal sensation that insects are crawling in the skin.

fourchette The back part of the female genitals at the entrance to the vagina.

four-day disease A lung disease of newborn infants, in which

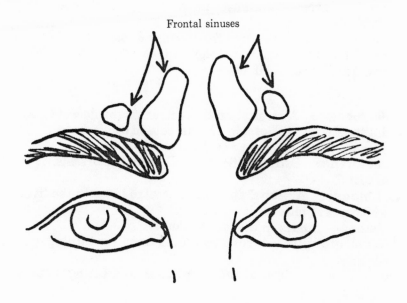

Frontal sinuses

The frontal sinuses.

the lungs become clogged with a membrane.

Fowler's solution A drug used in treating certain types of anemia.

foxglove The plant from which the drug *digitalis* is extracted.

fracture dislocation A dislocation accompanied by a fracture.

fragmentation Breaking into pieces.

F.R.C.P. Fellow of the Royal College of Physicians (British).

F.R.C.S. Fellow of the Royal College of Surgeons (British).

Friedman's test The rabbit test for pregnancy.

frigidity Lack of sexual desire in women.

Froehlich's syndrome A disturbance of the glandular system in which sexual organs remain undeveloped.

61

frontal sinuses The sinuses in the skull directly above the eyes.

frostbite A burn resulting from extreme cold.

funiculitis Inflammation of the cord leading to the testicle.

furuncle A small boil.

galactogogue A medication that increases the flow of milk.

galactocele A milk cyst in a breast caused by blockage of one or more of the mammary ducts.

galactorrhea Excessive flow of milk from the breasts.

gall Bile.

gall bladder A pear-shaped organ located beneath the liver which stores bile.

gallstones Stones in the gall bladder.

gamma globulin A chemical substance containing antibodies.

gamma ray A form of radiation, used in treating certain cancers.

ganglioma A tumor of nerve cells.

ganglion A cluster of nerve cells.

gangrene Death of body tissue.

Gantrisin Trademark for a sulfa drug used as a treatment against infection.

gargoylism Deformity of a newborn child.

gas gangrene A form of gangrene caused by a specific gas-forming germ which spreads through the muscles.

gastralgia Pain in the stomach.

gastrectomy The surgical removal of the whole or part of the stomach.

gastric Pertaining to the stomach.

gastric lavage Washing out the stomach.

gastric ulcer See *peptic ulcer*.

gastritis Inflammaton of the stomach wall.

gastrocnemius The main calf muscle in the back of the leg.

gastroenteritis Inflammation of the stomach and intestines.

gastroenterologist A physician who specializes in diseases of the stomach and intestinal tract.

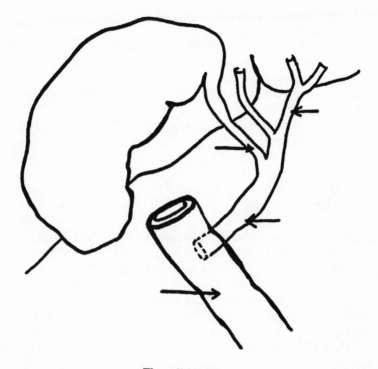

The gall bladder.

gastroenterostomy An operation in which the stomach is made to open directly into the small intestine in order to reroute the flow of food around an ulcer of the duodenum.

gastrointestinal Referring to the stomach and intestines.

gastroptosis A condition caused by downward displacement of the stomach.

gastrorrhaphy The repair of a stomach wound.

gastroscope A tube-like instrument for examining the inside of the stomach.

gastrostomy An operation to establish an artificial opening to the stomach.

gavage Forced feeding liquid directly into the stomach.

gel A mixture of liquid and solid which forms a semisolid substance.

gene The part of the chromosome which carries inherited characteristics.

general anesthesia Loss of sensation produced by administration of drugs.

generation Reproduction.

generic-named drug A drug that is sold under its technical name.

genetics The science dealing with heredity.

genitalia Sex organs.

genitourinary Referring to the sex organs and the urinary system.

genophobia An abnormal fear of sex.

genu The knee.

geratic Referring to old age.

geriatrics The science of medical care of old people.

germ A microorganism capable of producing disease.

German measles Rubella; a mild but highly infectious virus disease.

germicide Any substance that kills germs.

germinoma A tumor of the testicle (usually malignant).

gerontology The scientific study of the aged.

gestation The period that the infant spends in the mother's womb.

giant-cell tumor A type of tumor of the bone.

gibbosity Having a humped back.

gingiva The gums.

gingivectomy The surgical removal of a portion of the gums.

gingivitis An inflammation of the gums.

glands Any body organ which manufactures a liquid product that it secretes.

glandular fever Infectious mononucleosis characterized by sore throat, swollen glands, and weakness.

glandular tuberculosis Tuberculosis affecting the lymph nodes.

glans The head of the penis or the end of the clitoris.

glaucoma A disease of the eyes in which loss of vision is caused by fluid pressure inside the eyeball.

gleet Chronic gonorrhea.

glioblastoma A common type of brain tumor.

glomerate Rolled together like a ball of thread.

glomus tumor A vessel and nerve tumor, located beneath the skin or nails of the fingers or toes.

glossa The tongue.

glossalgia Pain in the tongue.

glossectomy Surgical removal of the tongue.

glossitis Inflammation of the tongue.

glossopharyngeal nerve The ninth cranial nerve supplying the tongue and throat.

glottis The two vocal cords and the space between them.

glucose Sugar in the form in which it usually appears in the blood stream.

glucose tolerance test A blood test for *diabetes mellitus*.

gluteus muscles The three muscles of the buttocks.

glycogenesis The formation of sugar in the liver.

glycosuria Sugar in the urine; frequently evidence of diabetes.

goiter An enlargement of the thyroid gland in the neck.

Goldblatt kidney A kidney to which the blood flow is reduced by disease.

gonad A sex gland.

gonadotropin A gonad-stimulating hormone.

gonagra Gout of the knee.

goniopuncture An operation to relieve glaucoma.

gonococcus The microbe which causes gonorrhea.

gonorrhea A contagious venereal disease, characterized by inflammation of the genital mucous membranes.

gouge A curved chisel used in cutting out portions of a bone.

gout A metabolic disease characterized by painful inflammation of the joints of the hands or feet.

GP General practitioner.

graft A tissue transplant.

grand mal A severe attack of epilepsy.

granulation tissue Newly formed tissue.

granulocyte A white blood cell.

granulocytopenia White blood cell disease.

granulosa-cell tumor A type of tumor of the ovary.

granuloma inguinale A chronic ulceration of the external sex organs.

gravel Small stones in the kidneys which is sometimes passed in the urine.

Graves' disease Another name for *exophthalmic goiter*.

gravid Pregnant.

grippe Influenza.

groin The area of the body where the legs meet the trunk.

growth hormone The hormone secreted by the pituitary gland at the base of the skull.

gumboil Abscess at the root of a decayed tooth.

gumma A rubbery growth that is one of the end results of syphilis.

gums The mucous membrane surrounding the teeth.

gut The intestine.

gynecologist A physician specializing in women's diseases.

gynecology The study of diseases in women.

gynecomastia Enlargement of the male breast.

gynoplasty Plastic surgery of the female genitalia.

habituation Drug addiction.

hair follicle The tiny sac from which a hair grows.

halitosis Bad breath.

hallucinogen Any substance that produces hallucinations.

hallux The great toe.

hamartoma A growth which is made up of excess growth of normal tissue cells.

hammer toe A toe which is bent and cannot be extended.

hamular Hook-shaped.

hand The part of the upper limb from the wrist to the finger tips.

Hand-Schüller-Christian disease See *xanthomatosis*.

Hanot's cirrhosis A form of cirrhosis of the liver.

Hansen's disease Leprosy.

haphalgesia A sensation of pain experienced when touching an object.

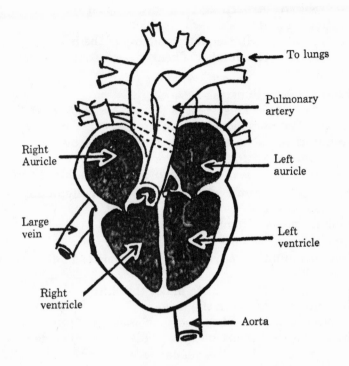

The heart.

haphephobia A fear of being touched or touching objects.

harelip A cleft in the upper lip.

hardening of the arteries See *arteriosclerosis*.

hay fever A swelling and watering of the nose and eyes, caused by allergy to various plant pollens, especially ragweed.

headache A pain in the head.

healing by first intention Normal healing of a stitched wound. (Also called *healing by primary union*.)

healing by second intention Healing without treatment.

heart The hollow muscular organ in the chest which pumps blood throughout the body.

heart beat The throb of the heart as it pumps blood.

heartburn   A burning pain in the upper abdomen or lower chest caused by stomach trouble.

heart failure   Inadequate pumping of the heart.

heart rate   The number of heart muscle contractions per minute.

heat stroke   Sunstroke.

heliotherapy   Treatment of disease by exposure to the sun.

helix   The rounded portion of the external ear.

helminthiases   Any disease caused by worms.

helotomy   Cutting out of a corn.

hemangioma   A non-malignant tumor of a blood vessel.

hemangiosarcoma   A malignant tumor stemming from a blood vessel.

hematemesis   Vomiting of blood.

hematic   Pertaining to blood.

hematologist   A physician who specializes in diseases of the blood.

hematoma   Hemorrhage under the skin.

hematuria   Blood in the urine.

hemicolectomy   The removal of one half of the large bowel.

hemicrania   Headache which appears on one side only.

hemiparesis   Paralysis of one side of the body.

hemodialysis   The separation of wastes or poisons from the circulating blood, by machine.

hemoglobin   The red coloring matter in blood cells which carries oxygen to the tissues.

hemolytic anemia   An anemia caused by the destruction of red blood cells.

hemophilia   A hereditary blood condition in which clotting does not occur normally.

hemoptysis   Coughing up blood.

hemorrhage   Bleeding.

hemorrhoidectomy   An operation for the cure of hemorrhoids.

hemorrhoids   Varicose veins of the anus which cause painful swellings.

hemospermia   Blood in the semen.

hemostasis A term indicating that the bleeding has been stopped.

hemostat An instrument for clamping a bleeding vein or artery.

hemotherapeutics Hemotherapy.

hemotherapy The use of blood in the treatment of a disease.

Henoch's purpura A children's disease characterized by bleeding beneath the skin usually accompanied by the appearance of "black and blue" marks.

hepar The liver.

hepar lobatum Syphilis of the liver.

heparin An anticoagulant given to prolong blood-clotting time.

hepatectomy The surgical removal of a part of the human liver.

hepatic Referring to the liver.

hepatic coma A state of unconsciousness evident in patients suffering from liver disease.

hepatitis Inflammation of the liver.

hepatoma Any tumor of the liver.

heredity The transmission of characteristics and tendencies of parents to their offspring.

hermaphrodite A person born with structures of both sexes.

hernia A rupture.

hernioplasty An operation for the cure of hernia.

herniorrhaphy An operation to repair a hernia.

herniotomy An operation to repair a hernia involving the opening of the sac of a hernia prior to repairing it.

heroin A narcotic related to morphine.

herpes simplex A virus infection, characterized by blisters or sores which appear in clusters about the lips.

heterotopia A deviation from natural position.

heterotoxin A poison originating outside the body.

heterotropia Cross-eye.

hexachlorophene A germicide.

hexadactylism Six fingers or toes.

hiatus hernia A type of hernia of the diaphragm.

hiccup A sudden spasm of the diaphragm.

hidrosis   Excessive perspiration.

hip   The joint where the thighbone and the pelvic bones meet.

Hippocratic oath   The oath sworn by a doctor: "I swear by Apollo Physician and Aesculapius and Hygeia and Panacea and all the gods and goddesses, making them my witnesses, that I will fulfill according to my ability and judgment this oath and covenant:

· "To hold him who has taught me this art as equal to my parents and to live my life in partnership with him, and if he is in need of money to give him a share of mine, and to regard his offspring as equal to my brothers in male lineage and to teach them this art—if they desire to learn it—without fee and covenant; to give a share of precepts and oral instruction and all the other learning to my sons and to the sons of him who has instructed me and to pupils who have signed the covenant and who have taken an oath according to the medical law, but to no one else.

"I will apply dietetic measures for the benefit of the sick according to my ability and judgment; I will keep them from harm and injustice.

"I will neither give a deadly drug to anybody if asked for it, nor will I make a suggestion to this effect. Similarly I will not give to a woman an abortive remedy. In purity and holiness I will guard my life and my art.

"I will not use the knife, not even on sufferers from stone, but will withdraw in favor of such men as are [skilled] in this work.

"Whatever houses I may visit, I will come for the benefit of the sick, remaining free of all intentional injustice, of all mischief and in particular of sexual relations with both male and female persons, be they free or slaves.

"What I may see or hear in the course of treatment or even outside of the treatment in regard to the life of men, which on no account [ought to be] spread abroad, I will keep to myself, holding such things shameful to be spoken about.

"If I fulfill this oath and do not violate it, may it be granted to me to enjoy life and art, being honored with fame among all men for all time to come; if I transgress it and swear falsely, may the opposite of all this be my lot."

histamine   A chemical substance occurring in human tissues.

histology   The study of cells and organs by microscope.

histoplasmosis   A fungus infection, sometimes erroniously diagnosed as tuberculosis.

hives   A condition in which whitish areas appear on the surface of the skin.

Hodgkin's disease   A malignant disease of the lymph nodes causing death.

homograft   A graft of tissue taken from the body of another person.

homolateral   Pertaining to the same side of the body.

homologous   Corresponding to the same type.

homosexuality   Sexual attraction toward one's own sex.

hookworm   An intestinal parasite.

hordeolum   An abscess on the eyelid.

hormone   A chemical produced by a gland affecting the function of another organ.

horseshoe kidney   A birth deformity in which the kidneys are fused in the shape of a horseshoe.

hot flashes   A sudden feeling of warmth, accompanied by sweating.

hourglass stomach   A stomach divided into two compartments.

housemaid's knee   A swelling below the knee caused by inflammation and fluid collection in the bursa.

Huhner's test   A female test for sterility.

humectant   A substance used to retain moisture.

humerus   The bone of the upper arm.

humor   Any body fluid.

humpback   A deformity of the spine.

hunchback   Humpback.

Hunner's ulcer   An ulcer of the urinary bladder.

Hunterian chancre   Syphilitic chancre.

Huntington's chorea   A disease of the central nervous system characterized by twitching muscles, an irregular walk, and poor speech.

Hutchinson's teeth A tooth deformity associated with inherited syphilis.

hyaline membrane disease A condition seen in newborn children in which a membrane covers the air sacs in the lungs.

hydatidiform mole A disease of the outer membranes of the uterus in which a mass of cysts develops.

hydatid of Morgagni A benign cyst occurring just above the testicle.

hydrargyria Mercury poisoning.

hydrarthrosis Fluid in a joint.

hydrocele An accumulation of fluid in a sac surrounding the testicle.

hydrocelectomy The removal of a hydrocele.

hydrocephalus An abnormal enlargement of an infant's head caused by an increase in the fluid inside the skull and commonly called "water on the brain."

hydrochloric acid An acid produced by the stomach.

hydrocortisone A cortisone medication.

hydrocyanic acid A poison.

hydromania Abnormal thirst.

hydromassage Massage by means of moving water.

hydronephrosis An excess accumulation of water in the kidney.

hydrophobia Rabies; fear of water.

hydrophthalmos Glaucoma.

hydrops The accumulation of fluid in body tissues or cavities. Dropsy.

hydrotherapy Treatment with water.

hydruria The elimination of urine in large quantities.

hygroscopic Readily absorbing moisture.

hymen The membrane covering the entrance to the vagina.

hymenotomy Cutting the maidenhead.

hyoid The U-shaped bone at the root of the tongue.

hypalgesia Insensitivity to pain.

hyperacidity Excess acid.

hyperactive child syndrome Minimal brain dysfunction.

hyperactivity Excessive or abnormal activity.

hyperalgesia Extreme sensitivity to pain.

hyperbaric oxygen treatment Treatment of disease by the administration of oxygen, under high pressure.

hyperchlorhydria Excess hydrochloric acid in the stomach.

hypercementosis Excessive cementum on the root of a tooth.

hypercholesterolemia An excess of cholesterol in the blood.

hyperchromatism Excess pigmentation.

hypercryalgesia Unusual sensitivity to cold.

hyperemesis Excessive vomiting.

hyperemesis gravidarum Nervous vomiting during pregnancy.

hyperemia An excess amount of blood in any part of the body.

hyperesthesia Excess sensitivity.

hyperglycemia Excessive sugar in the blood, as seen in *diabetes mellitus*.

hypergonadism Excessive secretion of hormones by the ovaries or testicles.

hyperhidrosis Excess sweating.

hyperinsulinism Insulin shock from an overdose of insulin; too much insulin secreted by the pancreas.

hyperkinetic Excess movement of muscles.

hyperlipemia Too much fat in the blood.

hypermania An advanced type of manic-depressive illness.

hypermastia Overgrowth of the breasts.

hypermetropia Farsightedness.

hypernephroma A type of tumor of the kidney.

hyperopia Farsightedness.

hyperosmia An acute sense of smell.

hyperperistalsis Overcontraction of the intestines, leading to diarrhea.

hyperpiesio High blood pressure.

hyperplasia Excess growth of cells.

hyperpotassemia Excess potassium in the blood.

hyperpyrexia High fever.

hypersalivation The secretion of too much saliva.

hypertension High blood pressure.

hyperthermalgesia Abnormal sensitivity to heat.

hyperthyroidism Overactivity of the thyroid gland.

hypertrichosis Excessive growth of hair.

hypertrophy Disproportionate growth of any organ of the body.

hyperventilation Abnormal deep breathing.

hyphemia A hemorrhage in the eyeball.

hypnalgia Pain occurring during sleep.

hypnoanalysis A form of psychotherapy combining psycho-analytic techniques with hypnosis.

hypnology The science dealing with sleep and hypnotism.

hypnotic Any drug that induces sleep, or that produces the effects ascribed to hypnotism.

hypnotize To bring into a state of hypnosis.

hypo Short for *hypodermic syringe* for giving an injection under the skin.

hypoacidity Deficiency of acid.

hypoagnathus An individual with no lower jaw.

hypobaropathy Altitude sickness.

hypocalcemia Too little calcium in the blood.

hypochlorhydria Too little hydrochloric acid in the stomach.

hypochondriac One who thinks he is afflicted with diseases which are not present.

hypodermic Beneath the skin.

hypofunction Decreased function.

hypogastrium Pubic region.

hypogenesis Underdevelopment.

hypogenitalism Underdevelopment of the sex organs.

hypogeusia Lessened sense of taste.

hypoglossal Under the tongue.

hypoglycemia Too little sugar in the blood.

hypogonadism Decreased function of the sex glands.

hypoinsulinism Diminished secretion of insulin by the pan-creas.

hypokalemia Too little potassium in the blood.

hypoleydigism Retarded sexual development.

hypomenorrhea Sparse menstrual flow.

hypoparathyroidism Inadequate function of the parathyroid glands.

hypoperfusion Reduction of blood flow through a part of the body.

hypophysectomy The surgical removal of the pituitary gland.

hypophysis The pituitary gland.

hypopituitarism Insufficient secretion of pituitary hormones.

hypoplasia Underdevelopment of an organ or tissue.

hyposensitivity Sluggish reaction to stimulation.

hyposmia Diminished sense of smell.

hypotension Low blood pressure.

hypothalamus A part of the brain below the cerebrum.

hypothermia A lower than normal body temperature.

hypothyroidism Underactivity of the thyroid gland.

hypotonia Poor muscle tone.

hypovitaminosis Deficiency of one or more vitamins in the diet.

hypovolemic shock Shock caused by loss of blood.

hysterectomy The surgical removal of the uterus.

hysterogram An X-ray of the uterus.

hysterotrachelectomy The surgical removal of the cervix.

iatrogenic Caused by the doctor.

ICCU Short for *intensive cardiac care unit.*

ichthyosis A disorder of the skin characterized by dryness and extreme scaliness commonly called "fish skin disease."

ichor A discharge from an ulcer or wound.

icterus See *jaundice.*

ICU Short for *intensive care unit.*

idiocy The lowest grade of mental deficiency.

idiopathic Of unknown cause.

idiot The lowest classification of feeble-mindedness.

ileitis Inflammation of the lower part of the small bowel.

ileocolitis Inflammation of both small and large intestines.

ileoproctostomy An operation in which the small intestine is stitched to the rectum.

ileosigmoidostomy A surgical procedure in which the small bowel is stitched to the sigmoid colon of the large bowel.

ileostomy A surgical procedure in which the small bowel is constructed into an artificial anus.

ileotransversostomy or **ileotransverse colostomy** An operation in which the lower part of the small intestine is connected to the transverse colon of the large bowel.

ileum The lower portion of the small intestine, ending in the large intestine.

ileus Obstruction of the small intestine.

iliac Pertaining to the ilium.

iliolumbar Referring to the muscles in the mid and lower back regions.

ilium The upper portion of the hipbone.

illuminism A mental condition in which the person imagines that he receives messages from supernatural beings.

imbecile A classification of feeble-mindedness one grade above idiot.

imbricate To close a wound with overlapping layers of tissue surgically.

immunity Protection against disease.

immunization Vaccination; providing immunity against diseases.

immunologist A physician who specializes in the study of immunity.

immunotransfusion A blood transfusion from a donor who is immune to the disease with which the recipient is afflicted.

impacted Firmly wedged-in, as an impacted wisdom tooth.

impacted cerumen Ear wax which has hardened.

impacted feces Stool which has hardened in the rectum and cannot be expelled naturally.

impacted wisdom tooth A third molar which is lying on its side, pressing against the second molar and cannot emerge normally.

impalpable Not capable of being felt with the hands.

imperforate Lacking a normal opening, such as an imperforate anus.

impetigo ˙A rapidly spreading, highly contagious skin infection characterized by red spots.

implant A tissue graft.

impotence Inability to maintain an erection of the penis.

impregnate To make pregnant.

inanition The physical condition resulting from starvation.

inbred Born to closely related parents.

incarcerated hernia A hernia in which the herniated parts are stuck in the hernia sac.

incise To cut.

incision A surgical cut.

incisor One of the four front cutting teeth of the upper and lower jaws.

inclination The tilt of an organ.

incompatible Substances which cannot be mixed with one another.

incontinence The inability to hold back urine or bowel movements.

incrustation Scab or scale.

incubation period The time required for a disease to develop after first contact.

incubus A nightmare.

incudectomy The surgical removal of the anvil bone in the middle ear.

indigestion Disturbed digestion.

induce To bring on; to cause.

induced labor Labor brought on by artificial means.

indwelling A tube or a catheter left inside an organ or duct to provide drainage, prevent obstruction, or maintain a path for administration of food or drugs.

inebriation Drunkenness.

infant Any child below the age of two years.

infantile paralysis Poliomyelitis.

infantile uterus An underdeveloped uterus in an adult.

infarct An area of dead or damaged tissue.

infection The existence of germs, viruses or parasites within the body.

infectious disease A disease caused by germs, fungi, or protozoa.

infectious hepatitis Inflammation of the liver caused by a virus.

infectious mononucleosis Glandular fever characterized by a sore throat, swollen glands, and weakness.

infecundity Sterility.

inflammation A reaction of the tissues to injury characterized by redness, heat, swelling, and pain.

inflammatory carcinoma A cancer associated with inflammation.

influenza Flu; a virus infection of the upper respiratory system.

infracardiac Situated below or beneath the heart.

infraclavicular region The region below the collarbone.

infracostal The region below the ribs.

inframammary incision A surgical incision beneath the breast.

infrared Electromagnetic waves used to give deep heat to an injured part of the body.

infusion The injection of a solution beneath the skin.

infusion reaction Fever and chills following infusion.

ingest To eat.

inguinal Pertaining to the groin.

inguinal hernia A hernia through the inguinal canal.

inguinal glands The glands that carry lymph secretions in the groin.

inguinodynia Pain in the groin.

inhalant A medication which is administered by breathing in.

inherited Derived from the parents by genetic transmission.

injection Anything forced into the body through a needle.

inlay A mold set into a cavity in a tooth.

inlet The entrance to a cavity.

innervation The nerve supply to a part of the part.

innocuous Not harmful.

innominate The hipbone.

innoxious Innocuous.

inoculation The injecting a vaccine or other substance in order to foster immunity to a disease.

inoperable A term referring to a condition so far advanced that it cannot be helped by surgery.

inquest   A legal inquiry into the cause of a death.

insanity   The legal term for a mental disorder.

in situ   In its natural position.

insemination   Fertilization of an egg by a sperm.

insomnia   Inability to sleep.

insufflate   To blow air, vapor or powder into a part of the body.

insulin   A hormone produced in the pancreas.

insulin shock   Coma as a result of an overdosage of insulin.

interarticular   Between two joints.

intercostal   Between the ribs.

intercurrent disease   A disease occurring concurrently with another disease.

internist   A physician who specializes in internal medicine.

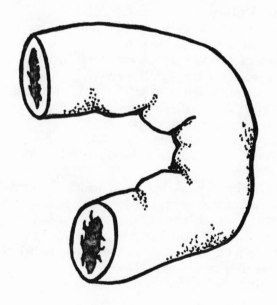

The intestine.

intertrigo An irritation of the skin caused by rubbing together two adjacent skin surfaces.

interventricular Between the two ventricles of the heart.

intestine The bowel.

intolerance Inability to take a specific medicine because of sensitivity.

intima The inner lining of the blood vessels.

intracranial Inside the skull.

intramedullary Within the bone marrow.

intrauterine Inside the uterus.

intrauterine life The life of the unborn child inside its mother's womb.

intrauterine transfusion A transfusion given to a fetus while it is within the womb.

intravenous Within a vein.

introitus The entrance to the vaginal canal.

in utero Unborn.

invasive Referring to a localized infection or tumor which *invades* other parts of the body.

inversion of the uterus A condition in which part of the uterus protrudes through the cervix.

ipecac A medication used to stimulate vomiting.

iridectomy The surgical removal of part of the iris.

iris The colored portion of the eye.

iritis Inflammation of the iris.

irradiation Treatment of a disease with radiation or radioactive substances.

irreducible hernia A hernia in which the contents of the hernia sac cannot be replaced in their normal position.

irrigation The washing out of wounds or body cavities.

ischemia Loss of blood supply to a particular part of the body.

islet-cell tumor A tumor in the pancreas which leads to hyperinsulinism and hypoglycemia.

I.U.D. Abbreviation for *intrauterine device*.

Jacksonian convulsion or seizure A form of epilepsy.

Jacksonian march A Jacksonian seizure which spreads to other parts of the body.

jail fever Typhus fever.

jalap A laxative.

jaundice A disease that causes the skin, eyes, and sometimes the mucous membranes to turn yellow.

jaws The bones which form the mouth. The upper jaw is the *maxilla*; the lower jaw is the *mandible*.

jejunal ulcer An ulcer located in the jejunum, the portion of the small intestine between the duodenum and ileum.

jejunitis Inflammation of the jejunum.

jejunojejunostomy The surgical creation of a passage between two loops of jejunum.

jejunostomy Surgical creation of an opening through the abdominal wall into the jejunum.

jejunum The upper part of the small intestine.

jiggers Sand fleas.

joint The place in which two or more connecting bones of the body fit together.

joint, Charcot's Arthritis of a joint, such as the knee, with swelling and loss of pain sensation.

jugular Pertaining to the jugular vein in the neck.

jugum A bridge.

junction The point where two or more structures come together.

jungle rot Any fungus infection of the skin originating from a trip to a tropical land.

juxtaposition Situated next to each other.

Kahn test A blood test for syphilis.

kala-azar An infectious tropical disease, transmitted by the bite of a sand fly.

kalemia Presence of potassium in the blood.

kangaroo tendon A tendon obtained from the tail of the kangaroo used for certain surgical sutures.

kaolin A smooth white powder used as a remedy for diarrhea.

Kaposi's disease A skin malignancy with marked pigment alteration.

karyotype The chromosome characteristics of an individual.

Keflin Trademark for *cephalothin*, an antibiotic.

keloids Overgrown scars which usually develop after surgery·

kenophobia A fear of empty spaces.

keratectomy The surgical excision of the cornea of the eye.

keratin The protein substance that is the chief constituent of hard body tissues as hair, nails, and the outer layer of the skin.

keratitis Inflammation of the cornea.

keratoacanthoma A skin tumor composed largely of hard keratin substance.

keratoconjunctivitis An inflammation of the cornea and conjunctival membranes.

keratoderma An inflammation of the skin, especially of the palms and soles.

keratoma Callus.

keratoplasty An operation for the transplantation of a portion of the cornea.

keratosis Any skin disease characterized by a thickening of the skin.

ketosis A type of *acidosis*, seen sometimes in severe diabetes.

kidney A bean-shaped organ lying high on the rear wall of the abdominal cavity which filters waste substances from the blood through the formation of urine.

kidney, arteriosclerotic A kidney in which there is hardening of the blood vessels.

kidney transplant An entire kidney transplanted from one individual to another, or from an animal to a human.

kinesia Airsickness, seasickness.

kinesiology The science which deals with human motion and particularly the coordinated action of brain, nerves, muscles, and limbs.

kinesthesia A sensitivity of the position of one's own limbs.

kinetics The science of motion.

kleptophobia A fear of thieves.

knee The joint between the thigh and the calf.

kneecap A disk-like bone in the front of the knee.

knit To heal, as a broken bone.

Kondoleon operation An operation for elephantitis in

82

which strips of skin, and tissue are removed by the surgeon.

Koplick spots   Spots in the mouth which portend measles.

Korsakoff's psychosis   A mental disease often caused by chronic alcoholism.

Kraske's operation   An operation for cancer of the rectum involving the removal of the rectum, part of the sacrum, and coccyx.

kraurosis   A dryness and atrophy of the skin or mucous membrane.

Krebiozen   An alleged cancer cure.

Krukenberg tumor   Cancer of the ovaries and pelvic organs.

kyllosis   Clubfoot.

kyphosis   Humpback.

The kidney

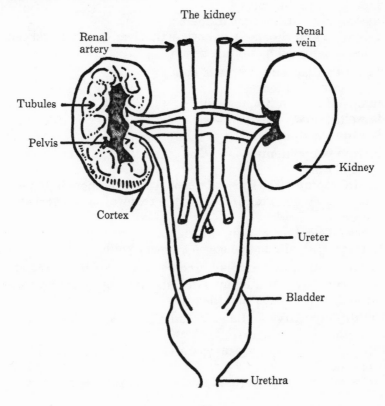

labia majora The major lips, or folds of skin, of the vagina.

labia minora Two thin skin folds next to the labia majora

labia oris The lips.

labia pudendi The lips of the vulva.

labor Childbirth.

labor pains The periodic pains caused by the contraction of the uterus.

labyrinth The maze of channels which make up the inner ear.

labyrinthitis Inflammation of the inner ear.

lac Milk.

laceration A wound made by a tear through the tissues.

lacrimation Crying.

lactation The secretion of milk from a mother's breasts.

lactose Milk sugar.

lactosuria Milk sugar in the urine.

Laennec's cirrhosis Cirrhosis of the liver with the liver cells being replaced by fibrous tissue.

Lafora's disease A type of epilepsy.

la grippe Influenza.

lame Having a limping gait.

lamella A thin plate or scale.

lamina A thin covering.

lamina propria mucosae The connective tissue of a mucous membrane.

laminectomy The surgical removal of one or more laminas of the vertebrae, often including the removal of the vertebral arch.

lance To cut or open by slitting.

lancet A small, double-edged surgical knife.

Landry-Guillain-Barré syndrome An infection of the spinal cord accompanied by paralysis starting in the legs and rising to the trunk and the arms.

Landry's paralysis Landry-Guillain-Barré syndrome.

lapactic Any laxative.

laparotomy Any surgical operation in which the abdomen is opened.

larkspur A medicine used against lice in the pubic hair.

laryngeal speech   Speech produced by means of an artificial larynx.

laryngectomy   The surgical removal of the voice box performed for cancer of the larnyx.

laryngitis   Inflammation of the larynx.

laryngoscope   An instrument with mirrors for looking into the larynx.

larynx   The voice box.

latent syphilis   Syphilis which remains in the body after the healing of primary and secondary lesions.

lateral   On the side.

lateral sinus thrombosis   A clot in the large vein of the lateral sinus in the skull.

latus   The flank.

laudanum   A tincture of 10% to 20% opium dissolved in alcohol.

laughing gas   Nitrous oxide, used as an inhalation anesthesia.

lavage   The washing out or irrigating of a body organ.

laxative   A medication given to gently move the bowels.

LD   Abbreviation for *lethal dose*.

lead anemia   Anemia resulting from lead poisoning.

lead poisoning   Poisoning caused by ingestion, inhalation, or absorption of damaging amounts of lead.

leather bottle stomach   Briton's disease. A thick-walled, leathery-appearing stomach caused by extensive cancer.

leech   An animal parasite which used to be used medically to suck blood from skin surfaces as a form of blood-letting.

Le Fort's operation   An operation for a "fallen womb" (prolapse of the uterus).

leg   The part of the lower limb between the knee and the ankle.

leiodermia (liodermia)   Abnormal smoothness and glossiness of the skin.

leiomyoma   A benign tumor composed of smooth muscle cells.·

lens   The portion of the eye behind the pupil.

lenticular astigmatism   Astigmatism due to defective curvature of the eye lens.

lentigo A dark brown spot on the skin of a person of middle age.

leper One afflicted with leprosy.

leprosy An infection generally occurring in tropical countries whose symptoms include loss of sensation and degeneration of parts of the body.

leptocephalus An individual with an abnormally small head.

leptomeninges The two main coverings of the brain and spinal cord.

lesbian A female homosexual.

lesion Any change in tissue structure due to injury or disease.

lethal Deadly.

lethal dose A dose sufficient to kill.

lethargic encephalitis Sleeping sickness tied in to an infection of the brain.

lethargy Stupor.

leukemia A group of malignant diseases of the white blood cells and blood-forming organs, sometimes called cancer of the blood.

leukocyte White blood cell.

leukocytosis An abnormal increase in the number of white blood cells which is usually a sign of infection.

leukoderma A condition in which patches of the skin have no pigment.

leukopenia A lower than normal number of white blood cells.

leukoplakia A disease, affecting middle-aged or elderly persons, characterized by white patches on the tongue, the inside of the cheeks and the gums.

leukorrhea A whitish discharge from the vagina, often caused by a fungus infection.

leukotomy Lobotomy. The surgical cutting of white nerve fibers in the front lobe of the brain.

levator ani muscle The chief muscle holding up the pelvic organs.

libido Sexual desire.

Librium Trademark for a tranquilizing drug.

lichenification Leathery hardening of the skin, often caused by irritation.

lien The spleen.

lienitis Inflammation of the spleen.

lienocele Hernia of the spleen.

ligaments Tough fibrous bands of tissue connecting bones at the joints and holding them in place.

ligamentum A ligament.

ligamentum flavum The connective tissue between the vertebrae.

ligamentum tarsi The ligaments of the ankle joint.

ligation The tying off of blood vessels during an operation.

ligature A thread or other material used to tie off a blood vessel.

lightening The slight sinking of the unborn child into the pelvic cavity during the middle of the ninth month of pregnancy.

lightning pains Severe, sharp pains coming on and disappearing rapidly.

limb An arm or leg.

liminal Threshold.

linear In a straight line.

liniment A liquid which is rubbed on the skin to loosen a muscle.

linitis plastica A type of extensive stomach cancer.

lipectomy The surgical removal of excess fat.

lipemia Excess fat in the blood.

lipid Fats and fatlike substances normally present in the body.

lipoma A nonmalignant, fatty tumor.

liposarcoma A malignant tumor originating from fat tissue.

lippitudo Inflammation of the eyelids; bleary-eyed.

lipuria Fat in the urine.

lithiasis The formation of stones.

lithotomy An operation for the removal of a stone, usually from the bladder.

litter A stretcher.

Little's disease Cerebral palsy in infants.

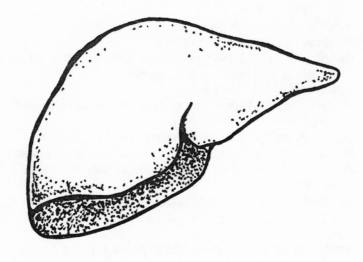

The liver.

liver The largest gland in the body, located just below the diaphragm and weighing 3 to 4 pounds.

liver spots Yellow and brownish discolorations on the skin.

livid A grayish-blue hue to the skin.

lobe The rounded part of an organ.

lobectomy Removal of a lobe by surgery.

lobotomy An operation in which part of the brain is removed in an attempt to alleviate a condition.

local Confined to an area.

localized Restricted to one spot or area in the body.

lochia The vaginal discharge that occurs in the early weeks after childbirth.

lock finger An affection of the fingers in which they suddenly become fixed in a bent position.

lockjaw Tetanus.

locomotor ataxia Syphilis of the spinal cord.

locus A spot.

logaphasia A brain disorder accompanied by an inability to speak.

loin The middle part of the back.

lordosis Swayback.

lotion Any liquid medication applied to the skin.

LSD Abbreviation for *lysergic acid diethylamide*, a hallucinatory drug.

lucid In full possession of one's senses.

lues Syphilis.

lumbago Lower back pain.

lumbar Pertaining to the loins.

lumbar puncture Spinal tap.

lumbar region The lower back.

lumen The space inside of a tube, as the blood vessel.

lungs The organs of breathing.

lupus erythematosus A skin disease marked by red scaly patches of various sizes on the skin which may affect the internal organs.

lupus vulgaris Tuberculosis of the skin.

luxation A dislocation.

lycorexia A very strong appetite.

lygophilia Love of dark places.

lymph The clear fluid found in the lymph vessels.

lymphadenectomy The removal of a lymph node.

lymphadenitis An inflammation of the lymph nodes.

lymphadenoma Enlargement of a lymph node caused by a tumor.

lymphadenopathy Any disease of lymph glands.

lymphangitis Inflammation of a lymph vessel.

lymphatic system A series of channels within the body which carry lymph.

lymphoblastoma A malignant tumor in the back of the nose and throat.

lymphogranuloma venereum A virus-produced disease usually spread by sexual contact.

lymphography   X-rays of lymph channels.

lymphoma   Any tumor composed of lymph node tissue.

lymphomatosis   See *Hodgkin's disease.*

lymphosarcoma   A malignant tumor of the lymph nodes or tissue.

lysergic acid diethylamide   See *LSD.*

lysin   A substance that can destroy living cells.

lysis   The receding of the symptoms of a disease.

McBurney's incision   A short diagonal incision in the right lower part of the abdomen, used in removing the appendix.

McBurney's point   A point of extreme tenderness in appendicitis where the appendix is usually located.

macerated   Softened as a result of being soaked.

macrodactyly   Abnormally large fingers or toes.

macroglossia   Enlargement of the tongue.

macromastia   Enlarged breasts.

macropsia   A disturbance of vision in which objects seem larger than they are.

macrosomia   Gigantism.

macule   A discolored spot on the skin.

madarosis   Loss of the eyelashes or eyebrows.

magma   Any pulpy mass.

magnesium   Milk of magnesia.

magnesium sulfate   Epsom salts.

maidenhead   The hymen.

major operation   Any potentially dangerous surgical operation.

major surgery   Major operation.

mal   Sickness, disease.

malady   An illness.

malaise   A feeling of being ill.

malaria   A parasitic disease transmitted by the bite of infected mosquitoes.

male climacteric   Change of life in the male.

malformation   A deformity.

malignancy   Cancer.

malignant Cancerous.

malignant glaucoma Glaucoma accompanied by violent pain rapidly leading to blindness.

malleable Easily molded.

malnutrition The state of being undernourished.

malocclusion A failure of the upper and lower teeth to meet properly.

malpractice Improper treatment.

Malta fever Undulant fever. A chronic infection caused by a germ often found in goat's milk.

malunion Poor or faulty healing of broken bones.

mammalgia Pain in a breast.

mammaplasty Plastic surgery upon a breast.

mammary Pertaining to the breast.

mammary glands The breasts.

mammilliplasty Plastic surgery of the nipple.

mammillitis Inflammation of the nipple.

mammography X-rays of the breast.

mandible The lower jawbone.

mania Excessive enthusiasm.

maniac An insane person with violent tendencies.

manic-depressive A form of insanity associated with alternating periods of great elation and great depression.

Mantoux test A skin test for tuberculosis.

manus The hand.

maple sugar urine disease An inherited disease, often ending in death, in which the infant's urine has the aroma of maple sugar.

marasmus Severe wasting of body tissues.

Marie-Strümpell encephalitis Arthritis associated with curvature and deformity of the spine.

marrow The soft, fatty tissues found inside the hollow spaces of the bones.

masochism An abnormal state in which one derives pleasure from receiving pain.

mass A lump.

mastalgia Pain in the breasts.

mastectomy An operation for removal of a breast.

91

masticate To chew.

mastitis Inflammation of the breast.

mastoid The breast-shaped bone of the skull, just behind the ear which is filled with air cells and which can become in fected.

mastoidectomy An operation for the removal of infected mastoid cells.

mastoiditis Inflammation of the mastoid cells.

mastoplasty Plastic surgery of the breasts.

masturbation Self-stimulation of the sexual organs.

maxilla The upper jaw bone.

maxillary sinus The sinus located in the cheekbone.

maxillofacial Pertaining to the lower half of the face.

Mazzini test A test for syphilis.

M.D. Doctor of Medicine.

M.D.S. Master of Dental Surgery.

measles A contagious virus disease characterized by inflammation of the mucous membranes of the eyes, nose, and throat, high fever and a typical rash.

meatus An opening or channel.

medial Toward the midline of the body.

mediastinitis Inflammation of the tissues in the *mediastinum*.

mediastinotomy The surgical formation of an opening into the *mediastinum*.

mediastinum The space beneath the breastbone containing the heart, aorta, trachea, and the other vessels and nerves of the area.

medicament A medication.

Mediterranean fever Malta fever.

medulla oblongata The part of the brain just above the beginning of the spinal cord.

medulla spinalis The spinal cord.

medulloblastoma A type of cancer of the brain, most common in children.

megacardia Enlargement of the heart.

megalomania A delusion of grandeur.

melalgia Pain in the arms or legs.

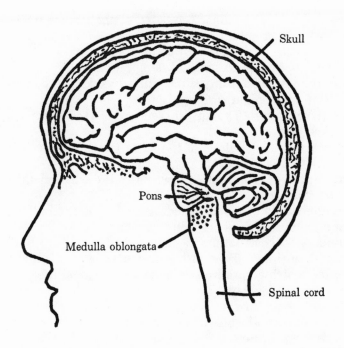

The medulla oblongata.

melancholia Severe mental depression.

melanoblastoma A malignant tumor of the skin stemming from pigment cells.

melanoma A cancer derived from cells containing pigment.

melena Dark, bloody feces.

melitis Inflammation of the cheek.

membrana tympani The eardrum.

membrane A thin layer of tissue.

menarche Onset of menstruation.

Ménière's disease A chronic disease characterized by dizziness, deafness, and noises in one or both ears.

meninges The three membranes that cover the brain and spinal cord.

meningioma A tumor composed of the tissues which cover the brain or spinal cord.

meningitis An inflammation of the meninges.

meningococcus A germ causing meningitis.

meningoencephalomyelitis Inflammation of the meninges, brain, and spinal cord at once.

meniscectomy The surgical removal of a torn cartilage in the knee joint.

meniscus A cartilage of the knee joint, frequently torn in athletic injuries.

menopause The time in a woman's life when menstruation ceases.

menorrhagia Profuse bleeding during menstruation.

menorrhea Excessive menstruation.

menses Menstruation.

menstruation The monthly discharge of blood from the vagina which occurs from puberty to change of life.

mensual Monthly.

mental retardation Arrested mental development.

menthol An alcohol made synthetically or derived from the oil of peppermint.

mephitic Foul.

meralgia Neuralgic pain in the thigh.

mercury A chemical used as a medication in combination with other substances.

meropia Partial blindness.

merosmia Partial loss of smell.

mesencephalon The middle portion of the brain.

mesentery The fold of tissue which connects the intestine with the back wall of the abdominal cavity.

mesial Towards the midline of the body.

mesosalpinx The connective tissue which surrounds the fallopian tube.

mesothelioma A tumor emanating from cells similar to those that line the abdominal chest and heart cavities.

metabolism The process by which foods are changed into basic elements to be used by the body for energy or growth.

metamorphosis A transformation.

Metaphen Trademark for *nitromersol*, a preparation useful as a local antiseptic.

metastasis Spread of a disease such as cancer within the body.

metatarsal Any one of the five long bones of the foot that reach from the ankle joint to the toes.

methadone A drug used as a substitute for heroin.

methyl alcohol Wood alcohol.

methyltestosterone An oral medication containing the male sex hormone.

methyltheobromine Caffeine.

metrapectic disease A disease passed along by a mother to a child which the mother herself does not possess.

metritis Inflammation of the lining of the uterus.

metrodynia Pain in the uterus.

metroptosis A prolapse of the uterus.

metrorrhagia Bleeding from the uterus between menstrual periods.

Meulengracht diet A high calorie, vitamin-rich diet sometimes prescribed for treatment of bleeding peptic ulcers.

microbes Germs.

microcephaly An abnormally small head.

microcyte An exceptionally small red blood cell.

microndontia Possessing an abnormally small tooth.

micromania A mental illness in which a patient imagines himself to be mentally or physically inferior.

microphotograph A photograph taken through a microscope.

microsurgery Surgery performed through a microscope, with special instruments.

micturition Urination.

midget A dwarf whose body proportions are normal.

migraine Severe headache often linked with spots before the eyes, nausea and vomiting. Generally, it is limited to one side of the head.

Mikulicz operation An operation for cancer of the large bowel.

Mikulicz's disease Overgrowth of a salivary gland in the neck.

milk crusts Scabs on the scalps of babies with eczema.

milk fever Fever occurring following childbirth caused by infection in the uterus.

milk leg A swollen leg resulting from phlebitis.

milk sugar Lactose.

milk teeth The baby teeth.

milk treatment The treatment of an ulcer of the stomach or duodenum by giving milk as the diet.

milphosis Baldness of the eyebrows.

Miltown Trademark for a popular tranquilizer drug.

minimal brain dysfunction syndrome A combination of learning and behavioral disabilities seen primarily in children of average intelligence.

minor operation An operation in which there is little danger to life.

miosis Contraction of the pupil of the eye.

miscarriage Expulsion of a dead fetus before the term of pregnancy is expired.

misogyny Hatred of women.

mitosis The division of living cells.

mitral commissurotomy An operation for the relief of mitral stenosis.

mitral stenosis Deformity of the mitral valve of the heart.

mitral valve The valve on the left side of the heart between the two heart chambers.

mobilize To free so as to be able to move.

molar One of the large back teeth.

mole A colored tumor of the skin.

molectomy The surgical removal of a mole.

monarthritis Arthritis affecting a single joint.

Mongolian idiocy Down's syndrome. A type of idiocy in which the child is born with an oblique slant of the eyes, like an Oriental's.

mongoloid Having physical characteristics associated with Down's syndrome.

moniliasis A fungus infection which may involve the mouth, skin, intestines, lungs, or vagina.

monobrachius An individual born with one arm.

monocyte A type of white blood cell having a single circular nucleus.

mononucleosis See *infectious mononucleosis*.

monoparesis Partial paralysis of an isolated part of the body.

monophagism Habitual eating of a single article of food.

monophobia Abnormal fear of being alone.

monoplegia Paralysis of a single limb or muscle.

monorchidism Being born with only one testicle.

monozygotic Developed from one egg.

mons veneris The slightly fatty pad over the female sex organ, covered with pubic hair.

Montgomery's glands Sweat glands in the nipple of the breast.

Moon's molars Deformity of the first molar teeth caused by inherited syphilis.

morbid Pertaining to disease.

morbidity rate The ratio of the number of sick people in a community to those who are healthy.

morbilli Measles.

morbus Disease.

morbus cucullaris Whooping cough.

morbus divinus Epilepsy.

morbus gallicus Syphilis.

morbus miseriae Any disease due to poverty.

morbus regius Jaundice.

mordacious Biting.

moria A dementia characterized by incoherent talkativeness.

morning sickness The nausea and vomiting that sometimes accompany women during the first months of pregnancy.

moron A mentally defective person with a mental age of between 7 and 12 years and an I.Q. of 50 to 69.

morphine A drug derived from opium used to relieve pain.

mors Death.

motility The ability to move.

motor Referring to any activity involving muscular movement.

motor alexia Loss of the ability to read aloud.

motor ataxia Inability to coordinate the muscles.

motor paralysis The loss of voluntary control of the skeletal muscle.

motor point A point on the skin over a muscle at which electric stimulation will cause contraction of the muscle.

M.R.C.P. Member of the Royal College of Physicians (British).

M.R.C.S. Member of the Royal College of Surgeons (British).

mucocele A cavity filled with mucous.

mucocolpos A collection of mucus in the vagina.

mucocutaneous junction The area where skin meets a mucous membrane.

mucoepidermoid tumor A tumor of the salivary glands.

mucopurulent Containing mucus mixed with pus.

mucosa Mucous membrane.

mucositis Inflammation of mucous membranes.

mucous Relating to mucus.

mucous membranes The lining of passages and cavities that lead from the inside of the body, come in contact with air, and secrete a fluid called mucus.

mucous vaginitis Vaginitis with a mucous secretion.

mucoviscidosis Cystic fibrosis of the pancreas.

mucus A thick liquid secreted by glands lining mucous membranes.

muliebria The female genitals.

Müllerian ducts Organs formed early in the female embryo that later become the fallopian tubes, uterus, and vagina.

multifamilial A disease affecting several successive generations of a family.

multilocular abscess An abscess containing many compartments.

multilocular cyst A cyst containing many compartments.

multimammae Having more than two breasts.

multipara A woman who has given birth to two or more children.

multiple myeloma A widespread disease of the bone marrow.

multiple sclerosis A chronic disease of the nervous system leading to partial paralyses and changes in speech.

mumps A contagious virus disease. .

mural Located in the wall of an organ

muriatic acid Hydrochloric acid.

murmur An abnormal heart beat.

muscarinism Mushroom poisoning.

muscle Tissue composed of fibers which have the ability to stretch and shorten, thereby causing bones and joints to move.

musculature The muscle system of the body.

musculoskeletal system The bones, muscles, ligaments, tendons and joints.

musicotherapy The use of music in the treatment of diseases.

mutilate To disfigure.

mutism Speechlessness.

myalgia Pain in the muscles.

myasthenia gravis A chronic disease of the nervous system, rendering the voluntary muscles exceedingly weak.

myatonia Lack of muscle tone.

mycetoma A chronic fungus infection.

mycobacteria Rod-shaped bacteria.

mycoid Resembling a fungus.

mycology The study of fungi.

mycosis Any infection caused by a fungus.

mydesis A discharge of pus from the eyelids.

mydriasis Dilation of the pupil of the eye.

myectomy The surgical removal of a muscle or part of a muscle.

myelic Pertaining to the spinal cord.

myelin The white, fatty substance that envelopes nerves.

myelitis Inflammation of the spinal cord or bone marrow.

myelocele Spina bifida, with protrusion of the spinal cord.

myelography X-ray of the spinal canal, carried out with the aid of an injected dye.

myeloid Pertaining to bone marrow.

myeloma Any malignant tumor of the bone marrow.

myelomalacia Softening of the spinal cord.

myelomeningitis Inflammation of the spinal cord and its meninges.

myeloparalysis Spinal paralysis.

myelopathy Any disease of the spinal cord or myeloid tissues.

myeloplegia Spinal paralysis.

myeloradiculitis Inflammation of the spinal cord and the roots of the spinal nerves.

myelorrhagia Bleeding of the spinal cord.

myelosclerosis Multiple sclerosis of the spinal cord.

myesthesia Being aware that one's own muscle is working.

myocardial infarction Damage to some part of heart muscle due to a loss of blood supply.

myocarditis Inflammation of the heart muscle.

myocardium Heart muscle.

myofascitis Inflammation of the muscle and coverings of muscle surrounding ligaments.

myography The recording of muscle movements.

myoma Benign tumor of muscle.

myomectomy Surgery which removes fibroids of the uterus.

myometrial hyperplasia Overgrowth of the muscle tissue of the uterus.

myometrium The muscle of the wall of the uterus.

myopia Nearsightedness.

myositis Inflammation of muscles.

myringitis Inflammation of the eardrum.

myringotomy Piercing the eardrum.

myxedema A metabolic disorder, usually due to degeneration or absence of the thyroid gland.

myxochondroma A benign tumor of the cartilage.

myxosarcoma A malignant tumor of connective tissue.

nabothian cyst A small cyst of the mucus glands present in the cervix.

nailing An operative procedure in which parts of a broken bone are held together by placing metal rods through them.

nails The flat, horny plates of tissue on the tips of the fingers and toes.

nanism Dwarfism.

nape The back of the neck.

narcissism Self-love.

narcolepsy A sleeping disorder characterized by uncontrollable attacks of drowsiness in the daytime.

narcosis A state of unconsciousness induced by a drug.

narcotic Any drug that produces sleep while relieving pain.

narcotism Narcotic addiction.

nares The nostrils.

nasal Pertaining to the nose.

nasopharyngitis Inflammation of the nose and throat.

nasopharynx The nose and throat.

nates The buttocks.

natural childbirth A form of childbirth in which a minimum of drugs is used.

nausea The feeling of being ready to vomit.

nearsightedness Myopia.

neck The part of the body between the head and the chest.

necromania A desire for death.

necrophilism Attraction to dead bodies; sexual intercourse with a corpse.

necrophobia A fear of dying.

necropsy Autopsy.

necrosis The death of body tissue.

Neisserian A polite term for gonorrhea.

nematodes Roundworms or threadworms.

Nembutal Trademark for a sleep inducing barbiturate.

neonatal Pertaining to a newborn infant.

neoplasm Any abnormal growth of body tissue such as a tumor.

neostigmine A drug used in the treatment of myasthenia gravis.

nephrectomy The surgical removal of a kidney.

nephritis Inflammation of the kidney.

nephrocarcinoma Cancer of the kidney.

nephrocystitis Inflammation of both the urinary bladder and kidney.

nephrolithotomy An operation for the removal of a stone from a kidney.

nephroma Any kidney tumor.

nephromegaly Kidney enlargement.

nephrosis Any degeneration of the kidney without inflammation.

nephrostomy An operation to form an opening leading to the pelvis of the kidney in order to drain the urine.

nerve The mechanism which transmits impulses and stimuli to and from the brain and spinal cord.

nerve block The interruption of the passage of impulses through a nerve, to produce loss of feeling to the area supplied by the nerve.

nerve deafness Deafness due to a lesion of the auditory nerve.

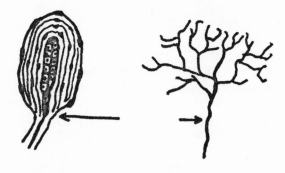

Two types of nerve structures.

nerve grafting The transplantation of a portion of a nerve.

nerve tract The path of a nerve.

neural Pertaining to nerves.

neuralgia Pain along the path of a nerve.

neurectomy The removal of a part of a nerve.

neuritis An inflammatory or degenerative condition of a nerve.

neuroblastoma A malignant tumor composed of primitive nerve tissue.

neurocalorimeter An instrument for measuring the heat of a nerve.

neurofibroma A nonmalignant tumor composed of nerve and fibrous tissues.

neurogenic Nervous.

neurologist A physician who concentrates on diseases of the nervous system.

neuroma A nerve tumor.

neuron A nerve cell.

neuropathy Any nervous disease.

neuroplasty A plastic operation on the nerves.

neuropsychiatrist A physician who specializes in both mental and nervous diseases.

neurosis An emotional disorder, without a severe accompanying personality change.

neurosurgeon A doctor who operates on the nervous system and the brain.

neurosurgery Surgery of the brain, spinal cord and nerves.

neurosyphilis Syphilis of any part of the nervous system.

neurotic An individual who is emotionally unstable.

neurotripsy The crushing of a nerve.

neutropenia White blood cell disease.

neutrophil A white blood cell.

nevus A mole or birthmark.

nevus pilosus A hairy mole.

nevus vasculosus Strawberry mark.

nictation The act of blinking.

nidus The center of infection.

Niemann-Pick disease A fatal hereditary disease affecting young children whose symptoms include the enlargement of the spleen and liver, anemia and mental deterioration.

NIH Abbreviation for *National Institutes of Health*.

niphablepsia Snow blindness.

nipple The point of outlet of the milk ducts of the breasts.

nitroglycerin A drug which dilates blood vessels and lowers blood pressure. It is used to relieve heart pain in attacks of angina pectoris.

nitrous oxide A short-acting anesthetic given by inhalation.

nocturia Getting up at night to urinate.

nocturnal Occurring during the night.

non compos mentis Not mentally responsible.

node Knotty localized swelling.

nonmalignant Not cancerous.

nose The organ of smell.

Novocain A trademark for *procaine hydrochloride*, a local anesthetic widely used in dentistry.

noxious Poisonous; harmful.

nucleus The living portion of a cell.

nucleus pulposus herniation A slipped disk.

nulliparous A female who has never borne a child.

nutriment Nourishment.

nyctalgia Pain occurring at night.

nyctalopia Night blindness.

nyctophobia Fear of the dark.

nymphomania Excessive sexual desire in a woman.

Oath of Hippocrates See *Hippocrates*.

obcecation or **obcaecation** Partial blindness.

obduction An autopsy.

obesity Overweight.

obstetrician A physician who specializes in delivering babies.

obstruction The state of being blocked.

obstruction, intestinal A condition in which the opening of the intestine is obstructed, either due to a growth within the intestines or by pressure from outside the bowel.

obstruction, ureteral Obstruction, often caused by a stone, of the path of urine from the kidney to the bladder.

obstruction, urinary Inability to pass urine from the bladder often associated with prostate trouble.

occiput The back of the head.

occlusion A closing or shutting off. Also, the fit of the teeth of the upper and lower jaws when the mouth is closed.

occult Concealed.

occult blood Blood which can only be detected by laboratory tests.

ochlophobia Fear of crowds.

ocular Pertaining to the eye.

oculist An ophthalmologist.

oculus caesius Glaucoma.

odontectomy The removal of a tooth.

odontoma A benign tumor stemming from a tooth.

odynacousis Pain caused by noises.

Ohara's disease See *tularemia*.

ointment A salve.

olecranon The funny bone; the tip end of the arm bone at the elbow.

olecranon bursitis Inflammation of the bursa of the elbow often accompanied by swelling and pus in the elbow region.

olfactory sense The sense of smell.

oligomenorrhea Infrequent menstruation.

oliguria Scanty urine.

omentectomy The surgical removal of the great omentum.

omentum A large membrane covering the lower part of the stomach.

omphalitis Inflammation of the navel.

onanism Masturbation.

oncology The science of tumors.

oncosis Any condition marked by the development of tumors.

onychia Inflammation of the bed of a nail.

onychophagist An individual addicted to biting his fingernails.

onychotomy An operation on a nail.

oophorectomy The surgical removal of an ovary.

oophoritis Inflammation of an ovary.

oophoron The ovary.

opaque Not transparent.

open chest cardiac massage Hand massage of the exposed heart.

open reduction Setting a broken bone by making a cut through the skin, exposing the broken ends, and bringing them into proper alignment.

operable A condition for which surgery is considered helpful.

operation Any surgical procedure.

ophthalmectomy Surgical removal of an eye.

ophthalmia Inflammation of the eye; conjunctivitis.

ophthalmologist A physician who specializes in diseases of the eye.

ophthalmamalacia Abnormal softness of the eye.

ophthalmophthisis Shrinking of the eyeball.

ophthalmoscope An instrument for examining the middle of the eye.

ophthalmotomy A surgical cut into the eye.

opiate Any narcotic derived from opium.

opsomania Intense craving for sweets.

optic Pertaining to the eye.

optician A technician who makes eyeglasses.

optic nerve The second cranial nerve connecting the retina of the eye with the brain.

optic neuritis Inflammation and sometimes degeneration of the optic nerve.

optometrist An individual licensed mainly to prescribe glasses.

oral Pertaining to the mouth.

orbit The bony socket containing the eye.

orchialgia Pain in the testicles.

orchiectomy The removal of one or both testicles.

orchitis Inflammation of the testicles.

organ A body structure which performs a specific function.

organic disease A disease associated with changes in the tissues of the body.

organism Any living body.

orgasm The climax of the sexual act.

orifice An opening to a body cavity or tube.

Orinase   Trademark for *tolbutamide*, an oral drug used in diabetes treatment.

ornithosis   A virus disease transmitted by parrots.

orofacial   Pertaining to the mouth and face.

orthodontia   The branch of dentistry concerned with deviation from normal alignment of the teeth.

orthodontist   A dentist who specializes in straightening teeth and correcting improper bites.

orthopedics   The branch of surgery concerned with deformities, diseases and conditions involving muscles, tendons, joints, ligaments, cartilage and bones.

orthopsychiatry   Preventive psychiatry.

orthoptics   Eye exercises.

os   A bone.

oscillation   Vibration.

osculate   To kiss.

Osgood-Schlatter disease   An inflammation of the tibia near the knee joint.

osmidrosis   Body odor.

osmosis   The passage of a substance through a membrane.

ossification   Formation of bone.

ostectomy   The surgical removal of a bone or a part of a bone.

osteitis   Bone inflammation.

osteitis deformans   Inflammation of the bones accompanied by marked deformity and thickening.

osteitis fibrosa cystica   Inflammation of the bones, with occasional cyst formation in bones.

osteoarthritis   Arthritis with bone and cartilage deterioration.

osteochondritis   Inflammation of a bone and its cartilage.

osteochondritis deformans juvenilis   Osteochondrosis of the head of the femur.

osteochondroma   A benign tumor of bone and cartilage.

osteochondrosis   Degeneration of bone growth localities in the bone of rapidly growing children.

osteoclasis   A surgical procedure in which a long bone is broken so that it can be reset more favorably.

osteogenic sarcoma   A highly malignant bone tumor.

osteoma A nonmalignant bone tumor.

osteomalacia Softening of the bones.

osteomyelitis Inflammation of the bone and bone-marrow cavity.

osteopathy Treatment of disease by manipulation of bones, joints, and other body tissues.

osteoporosis Over-porous bones.

osteosclerosis Abnormal hardening of the bones.

otalgia Earache.

otitis Inflammation of the ear.

otitis media Inflammation of the middle ear.

otitis sclerotica Inflammation of the inner ear accompanied by hardening of the tissues.

otolaryngologist A physician concerned with diseases and disorders of the ears, nose, and throat.

otoplasty Plastic surgery of the external ear.

otosclerosis Formation of spongy bone in the inner ear sometimes causing deafness.

ovarian agenesis Failure of the ovaries to develop.

ovarian pain Uterine pain sometimes following childbirth or abortion.

ovariectomy Removal of an ovary.

ovary The female reproductive gland, one on each side of the uterus.

oviducts The tubes through which the eggs travel from the ovaries to the womb.

ovulation The process during which an egg matures and is released from the ovary.

ovum The human egg.

oxygen tent An airtight chamber, enclosing the patient's head and shoulders, in which the oxygen level can be maintained at medically required pressure.

oxyopia Sharp vision.

oxytetracycline (Terramycin) A powerful antibiotic.

oxytocic Any drug that stimulates uterine contractions.

oxyuriasis Invasion by the threadworm or pinworm.

oz. Abbreviation for *ounce*.

ozena A disease in which the nose gives off a foul odor.

ozone   A form of oxygen.

ozostomia   Bad breath.

pachydermia   Thickening of the skin; "elephant skin."

pachyglossia   An abnormal thickness of the tongue.

pachymeningitis   Inflammation of the membrane covering the brain.

pack   A dressing placed on or around a part of the body.

Paget's disease   A chronic disease of the bones in which the skull, limbs and spine become thick and soft.

pagoplexia   Frostbite.

pain   Hurt.

painter's colic   Lead poisoning.

pain threshold   The point at which someone can no longer tolerate pain.

palate   The roof of the mouth.

palatitis   Inflammation of the palate.

palatoplasty   An operation to repair a cleft palate.

palliative   Any drug or treatment that relieves a condition but does not cure it.

palliative operation   An operation to make the patient more comfortable.

pallidectomy   The surgical destruction of ganglion cells in the thalamus to alleviate Parkinson's disease.

pallor   Paleness.

palpable   To be able to be felt.

palpation   Examination by feeling.

palpebra   Eyelid.

palpitation   Feeling one's own heart beat.

palsy   Paralysis.

panacea   A cure-all.

panarthritis   Inflammation of several joints simultaneously.

pancarditis   Inflammation of the heart.

Pancoast's tumor   A type of malignant lung tumor.

pancreas   A large gland located behind the lower part of the stomach which secretes enzymes into the intestines for digestion and manufactures insulin.

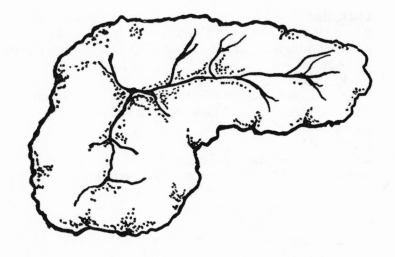

The pancreas.

pancreatis diabetes *Diabetes mellitus.*
pancreatic duct The tube which carries the secretions of the pancreas into the small intestine.
pancreatitis Inflammation of the pancreas.
pancreatolith A stone in the pancreas.
pancreatolithotomy The surgical removal of a stone from the pancreas.
pandemic disease A disease occurring extensively.
panhysterectomy Surgical removal of the uterus including the cervix.
panhysterocolpectomy Complete surgical removal of the uterus and vagina.
panniculitis Inflammation of the fat beneath the skin on the abdomen.

panophthalmitis Inflammation of all the structures of the eye.

pansinusitis Inflammation of all the sinuses.

pantaphobia The absence of fear.

pantothenic acid A part of the vitamin B complex.

Papanicolaou test or **smear** The "Pap smear;" a vaginal test for cancer in which the vagina and cervix of the uterus are swabbed with cotton and the cells are examined under a microscope.

papaverine A narcotic drug which relaxes muscles.

papilla A small, nipple-like growth.

papillitis Inflammation of the optic nerve.

papilloma Tumor-like growths.

papule A pimple.

paracentesis A puncture of any body cavity with a hollow needle to remove fluids.

paracme The period during which a disease remits.

paracolitis Inflammation of the tissue adjacent to the colon.

paracolpitis Inflammation of the connective tissue of the vagina.

paracyesis Extrauterine pregnancy.

paraglossia Inflammation of the muscles and connective tissues under the tongue.

paraldehyde A powerful hypnotic drug, often used to calm acute alcoholics.

paralogia Inability to think logically.

paralysis Loss of muscle function caused by injury to nerves which control them.

paralysis agitans Parkinson's disease.

paralyssa Rabies caused by the bite of a rabid bat.

paralytic One who is paralyzed.

paramenia Difficult menstruation.

parametritis Inflammation of the tissues surrounding the uterus.

paranasal sinuses Sinuses located around the nose.

paranoia A psychosis characterized by delusions of persecution, often accompanied by hallucinations.

paraplegia Paralysis of both legs, the result of severe injury to the spine or spinal cord.

paregoric A medication used to stop diarrhea.

parapsychology The study of psychic phenomena such as mental telepathy, and clairvoyance.

parasexuality Any sex perversion.

parathormone The hormone secreted by the parathyroid glands.

parathyroid glands Four small endocrine glands attached to the back of the thyroid gland in the neck. They secrete the hormone which controls calcium and phosphorus metabolism.

parathyroidectomy The removal of the parathyroid gland.

paratrichosis A condition in which the hair grows in abnormal places.

paregoric A medication used to stop diarrhea.

parenchyma The functional part of a body organ.

paresis Partial paralysis.

pareunia Sexual intercourse.

Parkinson's disease A degenerative disease of the nervous system involving a rhythmic tremor, rigidity of muscle action and slowing of all body motion.

paranychia A pus-containing inflammation around a nail.

parotid glands The saliva-producing glands in the back of the mouth, below the ear.

parotitis Inflammation of the parotid gland.

parous Referring to a woman who has had at least one child.

paroxysm A spasm, convulsion, or seizure.

parrot fever See *psittacosis*.

Parry's disease A name given to toxic goiter.

parturition Childbirth.

patch test An allergy test in which a small patch of adhesive containing a substance to which a person may be sensitive is applied to the skin and inspected a day or two later for reactions.

patella The kneecap.

pathogen Any agent which is capable of causing disease.

pathogenesis The course of the development of a disease.

pathologic Pertaining to disease.

pathologic fracture A break in the bone that occurs at the site of a disease in a bone without external causes.

pathologic lying (mendacity) Habitual lying.

pathologist A person who specializes in the study of the nature of disease by examining the tissues involved under the microscope.

pathology A study of the nature of disease based on an examination of the tissues involved.

Paul-Bunnell test A test for infectious mononucleosis.

P.D. Doctor of Pharmacy.

pectoral Pertaining to the chest or breast.

pederasty Anal intercourse between a man and a boy.

pedialgia Pain in the foot.

pediatrician A physician who specializes in diseases of children.

pedicular Infested with lice.

pediculosis A skin disease caused by lice.

pediculosis capitis Lice of the head.

pediculosis corporis Lice of the body.

pediculosis pubis Pubic-hair lice.

pedopathy Any disease of the foot.

pelage The hairy part of the body.

pellagra A common dietary deficiency disease whose symptoms include ulcers in the mouth, skin eruptions, diarrhea, and mental depression.

pelvic Pertaining to the pelvis.

pelvis A ring of bones at the base of the trunk, joining the spine and the legs.

pelvisection The surgical cutting of one or more of the pelvic bones.

pemphigus An acute or chronic skin disease, characterized by the formation of large blisters, and areas of skin slough.

penicillin The first and one of the most widely used antibiotics.

penis The male sex organ.

Penrose drain A rubber tube with gauze in its center inserted into the wound to drain pus and blood.

peptic Referring to digestion.

peptic ulcer   An ulcer of the stomach, duodenum or lower end of the esophagus.

percussion   Tapping parts of the body lightly with a hammer or the fingers and listening carefully to the sounds produced as an aid to diagnosis.

percutaneous   Performed through the skin, as an injection.

perforate   To pierce through.

perforated ulcer   An ulcer which has broken through the structure that houses it.

periadenitis   Inflammation of the tissues around a gland.

periarteritis   Inflammation of the outer layers of an artery and the tissues surrounding it.

periarteritis nodosa   A rare, often fatal, disease affecting arteries.

periarthritis   Inflammation of the tissues surrounding a joint.

pericarditis   An acute or chronic inflammation of the sheath which covers the heart.

pericardium   The sheath of tissue enveloping the heart.

perichondritis   Inflammation around the cartilage of a joint.

perihepatitis   Inflammation of the peritoneum and tissues surrounding the liver.

perimetritis   Inflammation of the tissues surrounding the uterus.

perimyositis   Inflammation of the connective tissues around a muscle.

perinatal   Referring to the time just preceding and immediately following birth.

perineoplasty   An operation to repair the tissue between the vagina and rectum which is often torn during a difficult childbirth.

perinephric abscess   An abscess in the area surrounding a kidney.

perinephritis   Inflammation of the tissues surrounding a kidney.

perineum   The part of the female body between the vagina and the anus.

periodontal   Surrounding a tooth.

periodontist A dentist who specializes in conditions which surround the teeth.

periosteum The elastic lining around bones.

periostitis Inflammation of the periosteum.

perionychia Inflammation around the nails.

periostosis Abnormal bone formation on the outside of a bone.

perisplenitis Inflammation of the covering of the spleen.

peritendinitis Inflammation of the sheath and tissues around a tendon.

peritoneum The membrane lining the interior of the abdominal cavity and holding the internal organs in place.

peritonitis Inflammation of the peritoneum.

peritonsillar abscess An abscess of the tonsil which has spread to the tissues surrounding it.

perivaginal Located around the vagina.

perivascular Near a blood vessel.

perle A capsule for easy administration of a liquid medication.

perlèche A mouth infection with grayish white patches.

pernicious Of intense severity.

pernicious anemia A type of anemia associated with lack of acid in the stomach and nervous disorders.

pernicious vomiting Vomiting during pregnancy which becomes so severe that it threatens life.

perodactylia Defective development of the fingers or toes.

peroral Passed through the mouth.

per os By the mouth, as the giving of a medicine.

per rectum Through the rectum.

Perthes' disease A children's bone disease involving inflammation of the head and neck of the thighbone.

pertussis Whooping cough.

pes A foot.

pes contortus Clubfoot.

pes planovalgus Flatfoot.

pes planus Flatfoot.

pessary An appliance used to help hold in place a prolapsed or displaced uterus, or to serve as a contraceptive.

pesticide A chemical used to kill lice and insects.

petechiae Tiny hemorrhages in the skin or mucous membranes.

petit mal A minor epileptic attack.

petrolatum Petroleum jelly.

peyote An intoxicating drug obtained from a Mexican cactus.

Peyronie's disease A disease of the shaft of the penis resulting in a deformity of the organ.

phacitis Inflammation of the lens of the eye.

phagocyte A white blood cell which can destroy foreign matter.

phagomania An uncontrollable desire for food.

phalacrosis Baldness.

phalanges The bones of the fingers or toes.

phalanx A bone of the fingers or toes.

phallic Pertaining to the penis.

phallus The penis.

phantasm An illusion or a hallucination.

phantom limb pain A sensation that a person feels in a limb which has been amputated.

phantom odontalgia Pain felt in the space from which a tooth has been extracted.

phantom tumor A swelling which looks like a tumor often caused by the contraction of a muscle or distention of the intestine.

pharmaceutical A medicinal drug.

pharmacist Druggist, apothecary.

pharmacology The science of medicines.

pharmacopeia A book that tells in exact detail how to make and use various types of drugs.

pharyngeal tonsil Adenoid.

pharyngitis Sore throat; inflammation of the pharynx.

pharyngoplegia Paralysis of the muscles of the pharynx.

pharyngorhinitis Inflammation of the nose and throat.

pharynx The area between the mouth and the opening of the esophagus; the throat.

phengophobia A fear of daylight.

phenobarbital A narcotic drug used in sleeping pills.

phenol A drug used as an antiseptic and disinfectant.

phenolphthalein A drug used as a laxative.

phenylketonuria PKU disease. Improper metabolism which causes infants to develop brain damage.

pheochromocytoma A tumor of the adrenal gland which may be accompanied by an increase in blood pressure.

Ph.G Graduate in Pharmacy.

phimosis A condition in which the foreskin cannot be pulled back over the head of the penis.

phlebectomy The excision of all or a part of a vein.

phlebitis Inflammation of a vein due to a clot.

phlebocarcinoma Cancer on the walls of a vein.

phlebolith A calcified deposit in a vein.

phlebophlebostomy An operation in which a connection is made between veins.

phleboplasty An operation for the repair of veins.

phlegm Thick mucus secreted from the lungs or bronchial tubes.

phlegmasia alba dolens A painful swelling of the leg often following childbirth.

phobia An abnormal fear.

phorotone An apparatus for exercising the eye muscles.

phosphorus A chemical which is a normal component of human blood.

phossy jaw Destruction of the jawbone common to people who fail to take proper precautions when working with phosphorus.

photodermatitis Any skin eruption caused by exposure to light.

photodynia Pain arising from over-intensive light.

photomania An abnormal desire for light.

photomicrograph A photograph taken through a microscope.

photophobia Abnormal fear of light.

phrenic Pertaining to the diaphragm.

phrenic nerves The nerves supplying the diaphragm which start in the neck and travel via the chest to the diaphragm.

phrenoplegia Paralysis of the diaphragm.

phthisis Tuberculosis.

physiatrics Physical medicine.

physic A laxative.

physical therapy The treatment of disease and injury by physical exercise.

physician One licensed to practice medicine.

physiognomy The physical shape of the face.

physiology The study of the function of living organisms.

physiotherapy Physical medicine.

phytosis Any disease caused by a vegetable parasite.

pia mater The membrane covering the brain and spinal cord and containing the blood vessels.

pica Craving for odd foods.

piebaldism Skin with areas lacking in pigment.

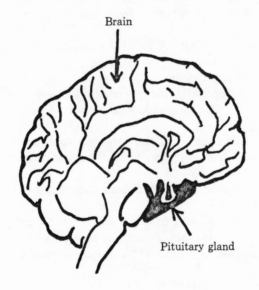

The pituitary gland.

pigeon breast or **chest** A chest with a deformity of the breastbone which makes it look like the breast of a pigeon.

pigeon-toed Walking with the toes turned in.

pigmentation Coloration of the skin.

piles Hemorrhoids.

pill A tablet containing medicine.

pilonidal cyst A cyst containing hair commonly found at the base of the spine.

pilosis Excessive growth of hair.

pimeluria Fat in the urine.

pimple A small pustule.

pineal gland A gland, about the size of a pea, located in the brain.

pinealoma A tumor of the pineal gland.

pinkeye. A contagious inflammation of the conjunctiva, a membrane which covers the inner surface of the eyelid.

pinna The outer ear.

pinworm A parasite which sometimes invades humans, causing inflammation of the bowel wall and rectal itching.

piptonychia Shedding of the nails.

pituitary The endocrine gland located at the base of the brain whose hormones regulate growth and control other endocrine glands.

pityriasis A skin disease marked by the presence of scales or flakes of skin.

pityriasis rosea An acute skin disease characterized by red patches over the body.

pityriasis rubra A serious skin disease involving the whole system. The skin turns deep red and is covered with white or gray scales.

PKU disease See *phenylketonuria*.

placebo A drug that looks like the real thing but has no medicinal value.

placenta Afterbirth. The structure in the uterus through which the fetus is fed.

placenta previa A placenta that is situated too low in the uterine cavity causing serious hemorrhage after the 28th week of pregnancy.

planing A procedure of cosmetic surgery in which skin is planed by sandpaper or a rotating steel-wire brush, to remove scars, pock marks, and superficial skin blemishes.

plantar warts Painful warts on the soles of the feet.

plasma The fluid part of the blood in which the blood cells are suspended.

plasmodium The parasite that causes malaria.

plaster of Paris A substance which is mixed with water and quickly hardens to form casts used in surgery.

plastic surgery Surgery which deals with repair of visible defects, scars and deformities.

platelets Small colorless disks in the blood essential to blood clotting.

platyhelminthes Tapeworms.

pledget A small, flattened compress of cotton or gauze.

plethora Excess of blood in the body.

pleura The membrane that covers the lungs and lines the inner walls of the chest cavity.

pleurisy Inflammation of the pleura.

pleuritis Pleurisy.

pleurodynia A severe, sudden pain in the side of the chest and along the ribs which disappears after a few days.

pleurotomy Incision into the pleura.

plexus A network of nerves or veins.

plica A fold of tissue.

plication Any surgical procedure in which folds are placed in a structure.

plug Material that blocks an opening or a duct.

plumbism Lead poisoning.

pluripara A woman who has given birth to several children.

pneumarthrosis Air or gas in a joint.

pneumatocardia Air or gas in the chambers of the heart.

pneumatometry The measurement of the pressure of inhaled and exhaled air.

pneumaturia Gas in the urine.

pneumocentesis Puncture of a lung with a needle to obtain material for diagnostic study.

pneumococcemia Blood poisoning caused by pneumococcus in the blood.

pneumococcus The germ which causes pneumonia.

pneumoconiasis Any disease of the lung caused by the inhalation of dust.

pneumohemothorax Air and blood in the chest cavity, sometimes the result of a stab wound of the chest.

pneumonectomy The surgical removal of an entire lung.

pneumonia An inflammation of one or both lungs.

pneumosclerosis Fibrosis of the lungs.

pneumothorax The accumulation of air or gas in the chest cavity.

pnigophobia A fear of choking.

podagra Gout.

podalgia Pain in the foot.

podalic Pertaining to the feet.

podalic version Changing the position of the baby inside the mother's womb so that it will be delivered feet first.

podedema Edema of the feet.

podiatrist A specialist in conditions affecting the feet; a Chiropodist.

podadynia A neuralgic pain in the heel of the foot without swelling or redness.

poison ivy An itching skin disorder resulting from contact with the poison ivy plant.

poison oak A plant which causes a skin condition similar to that from poison ivy.

poison sumac A smooth shrub which causes itch similar to that from poison ivy.

poker back or **spine** A stiff spine caused by arthritis of the vertebrae.

polio Poliomyelitis.

polioencephalitis Inflammation of the gray matter of the brain.

poliomyelitis Infantile paralysis.

Politzer's test A type of hearing test.

pollenosis Hay fever.

pollex The thumb.

121

polyarteritis Inflammation of several arteries.

polyarthritis Inflammation of several joints.

polychondritis Inflammation of cartilage in various parts of the body.

polyclinic A hospital in which many types of diseases are treated.

polycoria A hereditary deformity of the eye characterized by having more than one pupil.

polycystic kidney A kidney containing many cysts.

polycythemia A condition characterized by too many red blood cells.

polydactyly Having more than five fingers or toes.

polydipsia Excessive thirst.

polyhydramnios An excess of amniotic fluid during pregnancy.

polymastia Having more than two breasts.

polymorphic Occurring in several forms.

polymyositis Simultaneous inflammation of many muscles.

polyneuritis Inflammation of many nerves.

polyorexia Excessive hunger.

polyp A non-malignant tumor which hangs from the surface of a body cavity.

polypectomy The surgical removal of a polyp.

polyposis coli Multiple polyps of the large intestine.

pompholyx A skin disease characterized by blisters and peeling of the skin.

pons A bridge of tissue connecting two parts of an organ.

popliteal region The back of the knee.

pores The openings of the sweat glands in the skin.

porosis A bone condition in which calcium is replaced by cysts and soft tissue.

porphyria A metabolic defect. In certain individuals this condition may lead to abdominal colic, paralysis, mental disturbance, skin eruptions, and foul urine.

Porro's operation A cesarian childbirth immediately followed by a hysterectomy.

portal system The veins leading from the intestines to the liver.

portio vaginalis cervicis That portion of the cervix which extends into the vagina.

posterior In back of or behind.

posthemorrhagic Occurring after or resulting from a hemorrhage.

posthumous After death.

postictal Following a seizure or stroke.

postnatal The period immediately after birth.

postoperative After surgery.

postpartum Following childbirth.

postpartum hemorrhage A hemorrhage which occurs after childbirth.

postprandial After eating.

post-traumatic After an injury.

postvaccinal Following vaccination.

potable Fit to drink.

potassium An element normally found in the blood.

potency The ability of the male to have sexual intercourse.

potion A liquid medicine.

potomania Delirium tremens.

Pott's disease Tuberculosis of the spine.

Pott's fracture Fracture of the leg just above the ankle.

pouch A pocket.

poultice A soft mass applied to the skin for the purpose of increasing the blood supply to the area.

pox A small pimple containing pus.

prandial Pertaining to a meal.

preagonal Just before death.

preauricular In front of the ear.

precancerous Any tissue condition which may develop into cancer.

precipitate labor Sudden childbirth.

preclinical The course of a disease before it is diagnosed.

precocious Developing earlier than normally expected.

precordial pain Pain in the heart region.

precordium The chest area overlying the heart.

pre-eclampsia A toxic condition of pregnancy whose symptoms are high blood pressure, headache, abnormal weight gain, and swelling.

prefrontal lobotomy or **leukotomy** A form of psychosurgery on the brain used in treating certain types of mental illness.

pregnancy The period from conception to childbirth.

pregnancy test Any procedure used to diagnose pregnancy.

pregnancy, tubal Pregnancy developing in the fallopian tube.

pregnophobia A fear of becoming pregnant.

prelocomotion The movements of a child who has not yet learned to walk.

premalignant See *precancerous*.

premature Too soon, too early.

premature ejaculation Male ejaculation prior to or just after insertion of the penis into the vagina.

premature infant An infant born before the 37th week of pregnancy.

premature labor Labor taking place before its normal time.

premedication Administering drugs before anesthesia.

premenstrual Before menstruation.

prenatal Before birth.

prenatal care Care of the mother before giving childbirth.

preoperative Before an operation.

preoperative procedures Procedures to prepare a patient for surgery.

prepuce The foreskin of the penis.

presbyopia A form of farsightedness which comes with age.

presentation The position of the part of the fetus which emerges first from the cervix of the uterus.

presentation, breech The baby's buttocks and feet first.

presentation, cephalic The baby's head first.

presentation, face The baby's face first.

presentation, footling The baby's foot, or feet, first.

presentation, transverse The child lies crossways in the uterus and cannot be delivered unless this position is changed.

presentation, vertex The back of the baby's head first (the most common position).

preterminal Just before the end.

preventive medicine A branch of medicine which concerns itself with the prevention of disease.

priapism Constant erection of the penis without sexual desire.

prickly heat An inflammatory skin rash characterized by acute itching, brought on by heat and perspiration.

primary amputation An amputation performed immediately after injury.

primary shock Shock after an injury.

primigravida A woman who is pregnant for the first time.

primipara A woman who is delivering her first child or one who has borne one child.

p.r.n. A prescription abbreviation signifying *pro re nata* meaning "whenever necessary."

probe A slender metal rod used to explore wounds.

proboscis The nose.

procedure Any form of treatment.

procreate To produce children.

proctalgia Pain in the anus or rectum.

proctectomy The surgical removal of the anus and rectum.

proctoclysis Rectal feeding.

proctitis Inflammation of the anus and rectum.

proctologist A specialist in diseases of the anus and rectum.

proctoscope A hollow, metal tube inserted through the anus and rectum for the purpose of examination.

proctostomy An operation to establish a permanent artificial opening into the rectum.

prodrome A warning symptom of an oncoming disease.

progeria Premature aging.

progesterone The female sex hormone secreted by the ovaries.

prognosis The doctor's estimate of the outcome of a disease or injury.

progressive myopia of children Progressively worsening nearsightedness, due to growth of the eyeball.

prolapse The dropping of an internal body organ from its normal position. Most commonly, *prolapse of the uterus*, in

125

which the uterus protrudes into the vagina.

prolapsus ani The prolapse of the rectum, in which the rectum slips partially through the anus.

proliferation The rapid growth of tissue.

prone Lying face down.

propagate To reproduce.

prophylactic Any device that prevents the development of disease. Commonly used to describe the rubber sheath worn for the prevention of venereal disease.

prophylaxis Measures carried out to prevent disease.

proptosis Prolapse.

prostate The male gland behind the neck of the bladder which produces a fluid which is an important part of the semen.

prostatectomy The surgical removal of the prostate gland.

prostatism Enlargement of the prostate gland.

prostatitis Inflammation of the prostate gland.

prosthesis An artificial substitute for a missing part such as a tooth, hand or eye.

prosthodontics The replacement of missing dental and oral structures.

prosthodontist A dentist who specializes in prosthodontics.

prostration Complete exhaustion.

protein The principal component of the flesh of any living organism.

proteinuria The presence of protein in the urine, frequently an indication of kidney disease.

protoplasm Living matter.

protozoa The lowest form of animal life some of which cause human disease.

protuberance A knob-like projecting part.

proud flesh Overgrown tissue in a wound which has not yet healed.

provera A synthetic female hormone used to prevent spontaneous abortion.

provest A female oral contraceptive.

prurigo Chronic inflammation of the skin marked by severe itching and small papules.

pruritus Itching.

pruritus ani An itching in the anal area.

pruritus senilis Itching experienced by the aged, probably caused by a lack of oil in the skin.

pruritus vulvae Itching of the vulva and its surrounding parts.

psammoma A tumor of the membranes of the brain.

psellism Stuttering.

pseudoarthrosis A false joint.

pseudoappendicitis A condition simulating appendicitis.

pseudoblepsia A distorted image.

pseudocyesis False pregnancy.

pseudoedema A puffy condition simulating edema.

pseudohermaphrodite An individual who has the internal sex organs of one sex, but the external sex organs of the opposite sex.

pseudomania A mental disorder in which the person accuses himself of crimes of which he is innocent.

pseudomenstruation Bloody vaginal discharge in newborn girls.

pseudomucinous cystadenocarcinoma A cancer of the ovaries.

pseudopolyposis Warty growths of the lining of the intestines.

pseudopregnancy False pregnancy.

psittacosis Parrot fever; a severe, viral disease caused by a virus affecting parrots and other birds.

psomophagia Swallowing chunks of food without thorough chewing.

psoriasis An inflammatory skin disease in which reddish-brown areas appear on the skin which are soon covered with silvery-white or grayish scales.

psoriasis punctata A form of psoriasis in which the lesions consist of minute red papules which rapidly are replaced by pearly scales.

psychasthenia A nervous state characterized by an urge to think, feel, or do something senseless.

psychataxia Mental confusion.

psyche The mind.

psychedelic drugs Those whose actions seem to "expand the mind," such as LSD.

psychiatrist A physician who specializes in disorders of the mind.

psychic epilepsy A form of epilepsy in which the seizures are caused by an emotional experience.

psychoanalysis A method of treatment for some forms of mental illness.

psychogenic disorder Any illness of mental origin.

psychogenic headache Headache associated with tension, anxiety, or a basic personality disorder.

psychologist An individual trained in the science of psychology.

psychology The study of the mind.

psychoneurosis Neurosis.

psychopath A socially delinquent individual, not quite criminal and yet not normal.

psychopathic Pertaining to disturbed behavior.

psychosis A severe mental disorder, which manifests itself in abnormal behavior and reactions.

psychosomatic Imagined symptoms.

psychosurgery Treatment of mental illness with surgical procedures, such as lobotomy.

psychotherapy A method of treating mental disturbances.

psychotic Pertaining to psychosis.

psychrotherapy The treatment of disease by the application of cold.

pterygium A growth of mucous membrane tissue over the cornea of the eye.

ptilosis Loss of eyelashes.

ptomaine poisoning Food poisoning.

puberty The period of life when the sex organs begin to mature.

pudenda The external sex organs.

puerperal Referring to childbirth.

puerperal sepsis An acute infection of the genital tract following childbirth.

pulmonary   Pertaining to the lungs.

pulmonary embolism   The blocking of the pulmonary artery by an embolus.

purgative   Laxative.

purpura hemorrhagica   A condition caused by a below normal number of blood platelets.

purulent   Containing pus.

pus   The thick, creamy, yellowish liquid found in abscesses.

pustule   A small abscess, filled with pus.

pyelitis   Inflammation of the kidney.

pyelogram   An X-ray picture of the kidney.

pyelonephritis   Kidney infection, involving both the pelvis of the kidney and the kidney itself.

pyemia   Pus in the blood stream; blood poisoning.

pyorrhea   An inflammation of the gums around the teeth with pus formation.

pyrexia   Fever.

pyuria   Pus in the urine.

Q fever   An infectious disease caused by an organism associated with rickets. It can be caused by the bite of an infected tick or louse, by inhalation, handling infected material, or by drinking contaminated milk. Symptoms include: high fever, inflammation of the lungs, nausea and vomiting.

q.h.   A prescription abbreviation meaning *quaque hora*, every hour. "q 2 h" means "every two hours" etc.

q.i.d.   A prescription abbreviation meaning *quater in die*; four times daily.

q.l.   A prescription abbreviation meaning *quantum libet*; as much as is desired.

q.s.   A prescription abbreviation meaning *quantum satis*; as much as is necessary.

quadrant   A quarter of, such as the left lower quadrant of the abdomen.

quadriceps   The large muscles in the front of the thigh.

quadriplegia   Paralysis of both arms and both legs.

quarantine   The detaining and isolating of people who have been exposed to contagious diseases for a period of time equal to the longest incubation period of the disease to which they have been exposed.

quinine A drug extract, used in the treatment of malaria.

quinsy sore throat A sore throat caused by an abscess in the tissues around the tonsils.

quotidian An intermittent fever whose symptoms recur every day.

q.v. A prescription abbreviation meaning *quantum vis*; as much as is desired.

rabbit fever An infectious disease caused by a germ which gets into the body from handling infected rabbits.

rabid Having rabies (hydrophobia).

rabies A fatal virus disease, transmitted by infected animals.

rachiasmus Spasm of the muscles at the back of the neck.

rachis The spinal column.

rachitis Rickets.

radial Leading out from the center.

radiation burn A burn caused by exposure to X-ray or sunlight.

radiation carcinoma A cancer caused by overexposure to radiation.

radiation sickness Illness due to the effects of radiation therapy, usually characterized by nausea and vomiting.

radiation therapy Treatment with X-rays, radium, cobalt or other radioactive materials to destroy a tumor.

radical cesarean section Cesarean section immediately followed by a hysterectomy.

radical mastectomy The surgical removal of the entire breast and the adjacent tissue including some chest muscles.

radical surgery A massive attempt to eradicate a disease.

radical treatment Extensive treatment.

radiculitis Inflammation at the root of a nerve, especially one whose roots are in the spinal cord.

radioactive Referring to any substance which emits radiant energy, such as radium.

radiodermatitis Skin inflammation caused by radiation treatment.

radiography Taking and studying X-ray pictures

radiologist A physician specializing in radiology.

radiology The branch of medicine that deals with radioactive substances and their use in diagnosing and treating disease.

radiopaque A substance which can be detected by X-rays, such as barium.

radiosurgery The use of radium in surgical treatment.

radiotherapy Radiation therapy.

radiothermy Treatment by radiant heat; diathermy.

radium A radioactive metal used in the treatment of certain malignant diseases.

radium implantation A treatment for malignancy involving the placement of metal needles containing radium into tissues, allowing them to remain in place for a specified period of time before removing them.

radius The outer bone of the forearm.

radon The radioactive gas produced by radium used in treating malignant tumors.

radon seed A metal container for radon implanted in a malignant tumor to destroy it.

ragweed A weed whose pollen causes hay fever.

rale Any sound in the lungs that shouldn't be there and whose presence indicates that something is wrong.

ramus A branch of an artery, vein, nerve or bone.

ranula A cyst of a salivary gland, located beneath the tongue.

rat bite fever One of two diseases caused by the bite of an infected rat.

Raynaud's disease A disease often caused by a chronic constriction and spasm of the blood vessels in the fingers, toes, or tip of the nose.

reaction Response to stimulation.

reaction, immune A reaction to a test which shows that an individual has not contracted a certain disease.

reaction time The period which elapses between the stimulation and the response to it.

reagent Anything that causes a chemical reaction.

recessive characteristics Characteristics not visible when inherited.

recidivation Recurrence of an illness.

rectalgia Pain in the rectal area.

rectocele Extension of the rectum into the vagina associated with prolapse of the uterus.

rectocolitis Inflammation of the large bowel and rectum.

rectosigmoidectomy The surgical removal of the rectum and portions of the large intestine.

rectum The lower part of the large bowel, ending with the anus.

recumbent Lying down.

reducible hernia A hernia whose contents can be replaced through the opening of the hernia.

reduction When applied to a fracture, it means setting the fracture and bringing the broken sections into alignment.

reflex An involuntary act or movement performed in response to stimulus.

reflux A return flow.

refractory Not responding to treatment.

regeneration The formation of new tissues by the body after the old ones have been destroyed by disease or injury.

regimen A plan of treatment.

regional ileitis Inflammation in a region of the small intestine.

regression Reversion to earlier types of behavior.

regurgitation Vomiting.

reinfection A second infection from the same germ.

reinfection tuberculosis Chronic tuberculosis.

reinnervation Nerve grafting to restore nerve function.

rejuvenescence A restoration of sexual appetite.

relapse Getting sicker after having improved.

relapsing fever The name for a group of infectious diseases caused by a microbe characterized by recurring attacks of high fever.

REM *Rapid eye movement.*

remission The disappearance of symptoms of disease without the elimination of the cause of the disease.

renal Referring to the kidneys.

renal calculus A kidney stone.

renal-cell carcinoma A form of kidney cancer.

resect To cut out by surgery.

resection The operation of cutting out.

resident A physician serving in a hospital for further training.

resolution The clearing up of an infection.

resolve To return to a normal state.

respirator An iron lung; a machine which performs artificial respiration.

respiratory system The nose, throat, larynx, trachea, bronchial tubes and lungs.

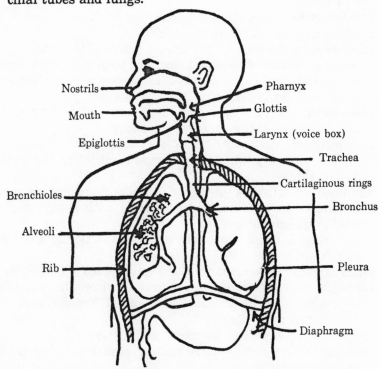

Nostrils
Mouth
Epiglottis
Bronchioles
Alveoli
Rib
Pharnyx
Glottis
Larynx (voice box)
Trachea
Cartilaginous rings
Bronchus
Pleura
Diaphragm

The respiratory system.

resuscitation Artificial respiration.

rete A network of nerves or blood vessels.

retching Vomiting without food returning from the stomach.

reticulocyte An immature red blood cell.

reticulum cell sarcoma A malignant tumor emanating from cells of the reticuloendothelial system.

retina The light-sensitive lining of the eye.

retinitis Inflammation of the retina.

retinoblastoma A malignant tumor of the retina.

retrobulbar neuritis Inflammation of the optic nerve.

retrodisplacement A term used to describe shifting of the uterus backward in the abdomen.

retrograde Moving in the wrong direction, as a retrograde flow of blood.

retrogression Degeneration.

rhabdomyoma A tumor of muscles.

rhabdomyosarcoma A malignant tumor of the muscle.

rheumatic fever A disease associated with high fever, painful swelling of the joints, and inflammation of the valves and muscles of the heart.

rheumatic heart disease Inflammation of the heart muscle and distortion of the valves of the heart.

rheumatism An overall term used to indicate diseases of muscle, tendon, joint, bone, or nerves resulting in discomfort and disability.

rheumatoid arthritis A type of arthritis characterized by an inflammation of joints and associated with symptoms resembling rheumatism.

Rh factor A blood component important in typing blood for transfusions.

rhinitis Any inflammation of the nasal mucous membrane.

rhinophyma A form of acne which results in swelling and the formation of large nodules. Also called "toper's nose" or "whiskey nose."

rhinoplasty A plastic operation on the nose.

rhizotomy Surgery to cut the roots of spinal nerves in order to relieve incurable pain.

rhonci Rattling in the throat.

rhythm method A method of preventing pregnancy by avoiding sexual intercourse during the time when ovulation is likely to occur.

rib   One of 24 bones forming the chest cage.

riboflavin   Vitamin B$_2$.

rickets   The twisted bone disorder due to lack of vitamin D in childhood.

Rickettsial diseases   A group of diseases caused by bacteria-like organisms including typhus fever, Q fever, and Rocky Mountain spotted fever.

Riedel's struma   An inflammatory disease of the thyroid gland.

rigor mortis   Stiffness of the muscles after death.

ringworm   A fungus infection of the skin so called because it spreads outward to form a ring.

R.N.   Registered Nurse.

Rocky Mountain spotted fever   An infection caused by the bite of an infected tick.

rodent ulcer   A common, curable skin cancer, seen most often on the faces of older people.

roentgen therapy   X-ray therapy.

Rokitansky's disease   Poisoning of the liver with rapid destruction of liver tissue. Also called *acute yellow atrophy* of the liver.

Rorschach test   A test of personality using inkblots.

rose fever   A form of hay fever.

roseqla infantum   A contagious childhood disease characterized by a fever followed by a light rose-colored rash and then a sudden drop in fever.

roughage   Food containing material which will not be easily digested.

round-cell carcinoma   A form of lung cancer.

round ligament of the liver   A band of tissue extending from the under side of the navel to the liver.

roundworm   A worm which sometimes invades the intestinal tract.

rubefacient   Anything that reddens the skin by bringing additional blood to it.

rubella   German measles; characterized by a light pink rash and swollen glands.

rubeola   Measles.

Rubin's test A test of the fallopian tubes to see if they can permit an ovum to pass. The test is carried out by injecting a gas into the cervix and viewing with X-rays.

rubor Redness caused by inflammation.

ructus Belching.

rudimentary Undeveloped.

rugitus Rumbling of the intestines.

rump The buttocks.

rupture A hernia; a tearing of a part.

rupture of the bag of water Same as rupture of the birth sac.

rupture of membranes A tear in the membrane surrounding the unborn child.

saber shin A thickening of the shinbone (tibia) caused by · syphilis or yaws.

Sabin vaccine An oral vaccine for the prevention of infantile paralysis.

sac Any pouch covering a body cavity, hernia, cyst or tumor.

saccharin A chemical substitute for sugar containing few calories.

sacralization A spinal deformity in which the fifth lumbar vertebra is fused to the sacrum.

sacrectomy The surgical removal of part of the sacrum.

sacrococcygeal region The area of the spine above the anus.

sacroiliac The joint between the sacrum and ilium (hipbone) and the ligaments that join them.

sacrum The last five vertebrae of the spinal column which form a triangular bone, which is the back wall of the pelvis.

sadism Sexual pleasure derived from hurting people.

sadist One who takes pleasure in hurting others.

Saint Agatha's disease Any disease of the female breast.

Saint Agnan's disease Ringworm.

Saint Aman's disease Pellagra.

Saint Anthony's fire An infection of the skin.

Saint Avertin's disease Epilepsy.

Saint Blaize's disease Quinsy.

Saint Erasmus' disease Colic.

Saint Fiacre's disease Hemorrhoids.

Saint Gervasius' disease Rheumatism.

Saint Giles' disease Leprosy.

Saint Gothard's disease Ancylostomiasis.

Saint Ignatius' itch Pellagra.

St. Louis encephalitis An infection of the central nervous system.

Saint Main's evil Scabies.

Saint Martin's disease Alcoholism.

Saint Roch's disease Bubonic plague.

Saint Sebastian's disease Plague.

Saint Valentine's disease Epilepsy.

Saint Vitus' dance A disease of the nerves characterized by unpredictable movements of the muscles of the limbs and face.

Saint Zachary's disease Mutism.

salicylate drugs Drugs that have the same general effects as aspirin.

saline solution Salt solution.

saliva Spit.

salivary glands The glands which produce and secrete saliva.

Salk vaccine Polio vaccine.

Salmonela A type of germ sometimes responsible for food poisoning.

salmonella fever A disease similar to typhoid fever.

salpingectomy The surgical excision of the fallopian tube.

salpingitis Inflammation of the fallopian tubes. Also, inflammation of the tube between the ear and throat.

salpingoplasty An operation to reopen a closed fallopian tube.

saltpeter Potassium nitrate.

salve Any ointment.

sanatorium An institution designed to treat people suffering from long-lasting illnesses or mental disorders but requiring constant medical care.

sanguine Bloody.

San Joaquin Valley fever A lung infection seen among residents of the San Joaquin Valley in California.

saphenous vein Either of the two veins of the leg and thigh which are near the surface of the skin and are usually involved in varicose veins.

sapphism Lesbianism; female homosexuality.

sarcoidosis A disease in which lumps and tumors appear on the skin.

sarcoma A cancer in a connective tissue.

sartorius The muscle in the thigh which enables one to cross one leg over the other.

saturnism Lead poisoning.

satyriasis Excessive sexual desire in the male.

scabies "Seven-year itch." A skin disorder caused by an insect which burrows under the skin and lays eggs.

scalenotomy Cutting the scalene muscles in the neck to relieve pressure exerted on the nerves going to the arm.

scalenus One of three muscles in the neck which emerge near the spinal vertebrae and extend to the front portion of the first two ribs.

scalp The skin covering the skull.

scalpel A short surgical knife with a curved blade.

scanning speech Slow speech with pauses between syllables caused by brain lesions and common in multiple sclerosis victims.

scaphoid Boat-shaped bones in the hands and feet.

scapula The shoulder blade.

scarlatina Scarlet fever.

scarlet fever An infectious disease characterized by a scarlet skin eruption. Symptoms include a painful sore throat, chill, nausea, vomiting, and high fever.

scatology The study of feces to diagnose disease.

scatophagy The eating of excrement.

Sc.D Doctor of Science.

Schick test A skin test to determine if one is immune to diphtheria.

Schilder's disease A disease of the brain and nerves leading from the brain.

schistorrhachis Spina bifida.

schistosomiasis A tropical disease caused by invasion of the *bilharzia* parasite.

schizoid Resembling schizophrenia.

schizophrenia A severe mental disorder in which a person withdraws from reality and suffers hallucinations, sometimes without loss of intelligence.

Schultz-Charlton test A skin test to determine if one is immune to scarlet fever.

sciatica A form of neuralgia causing pain along the sciatic nerve (which runs down the back of the thigh and into the leg).

sclera The white of the eye.

scleritis Inflammation of the white of the eye which may involve the cornea, iris, and choroid.

scleroderma A disease in which all the layers of the skin become rigid.

sclerosis Hardening of tissues.

scoliosis Abnormal curvature of the spine.

scopophobia Fear of being seen.

scotoma A blind spot on the retina.

scrofula Tuberculosis of the lymph glands.

scrotum The sack which contains the testicles.

scurvy A deficiency disease caused by a lack of vitamin C. Symptoms include weakness, spongy gums, and bleeding under the skin and from the mucous membranes and bone coverings.

sebaceous glands The glands of the skin which secrete sebum.

seborrheic dermatitis A skin disease caused by oversecretion of the sebaceous glands.

sebum The oily substance secreted by the sebaceous glands.

secondary infection The occurrence of a new infection upon an existing infection.

secondary sex characters Differences between males and females not concerned with reproduction, such as voice or hair.

second-look operation An operation performed on a cancer patient a few months after the initial operation to make sure that all the cancerous tissue was removed.

secreta Any substance which is secreted by a gland.

secrete To expel a substance in the way that the salivary glands secrete saliva.

sedative Any drug that calms the nerves.

seizure A sudden attack; an epileptic convulsion.

self-limited A term describing a disease which lasts a specific length of time and then disappears.

semen The male fertilizing fluid.

semicoma A state of partial or mild coma from which a patient can be aroused, though with difficulty.

semicomatose Being in a state of semicoma.

semiconscious Partially conscious.

semimenbranosus One of the "hamstring" muscles extending down the back of the thigh.

seminal vesicles The glands near the prostate and urethra which store semen prior to its ejaculation.

seminoma A malignant tumor of the testicles.

semitendinosus One of the "hamstring" muscles extending down the back of the thigh.

senectitude Old age.

senescence The process of aging.

senile Referring to unreliable behavior because of old age.

senile dementia A brain condition associated with old age, usually characterized by difficulties in assimilating new information and experiences, and mental deterioration.

senile involution The slowly progressive degenerative body changes seen with age.

senile psychosis A severe form of chronic brain disorder associated with old age characterized by personality deterioration, heavy memory loss, eccentricity, stubbornness, and often extreme irritability.

senility Old age.

senopia The change of vision in the aged in which persons formerly nearsighted acquire normal vision due to eye changes.

sensory Pertaining to sensation.

sepsis Poisoning by bacteria which circulate in the blood.

septic Infected.

septicemia Blood-poisoning, usually marked by high fever, sweating and prostration.

septic sore throat An acute infection of the throat caused by the streptococcus hemolyticus organism.

septum A wall between parts of the body.

septum nasi Nasal septum.

sequela An abnormal condition following a disease such as residual paralysis following acute paralytic polio.

sequestrum A small piece of dead bone that has broken loose from its base as a result of disease of the bone.

serology The branch of science which studies the serum of the blood.

seroma A collection of serum which produces a tumor-like swelling beneath the skin.

serositis An inflammation of a membrane lining the abdominal cavity.

serum The liquid part of the blood that remains when the solid elements in it have been removed by clotting.

serum sickness Illness following the injection of a serum into someone who is allergic to an ingredient in the serum.

sesamoid bones Small extra bones which develop in tendons.

sex chromosome The X and Y chromosomes, the chromosomes which determine the sex of an individual.

shaking palsy Parkinson's disease.

shank The leg from the knee to the ankle.

sheath The connective tissue covering an organ.

shigella A germ which causes diarrhea, dysentery, and other bowel ailments.

shigellosis Dysentery.

shinbone Tibia.

shingles Herpes zoster. A virus infection of the nerve endings in the skin characterized by the formation of blisters, crusts and severe pain.

shock A change of bodily state caused by a rapid fall in blood pressure following injury, operation or the administration of anesthesia.

shock therapy The treatment of psychiatric patients by passing an electric current through the brain.

shot A popular term denoting an injection or inoculation.

shoulder The region where the arm joins the body.

shunt A bypass.

sialoadenectomy The surgical removal of a salivary gland.

sialodenitis Inflammation of a salivary gland.

sialorrhea Flow of saliva.

sicchasia Nausea.

sickle cell anemia A type of anemia seen mostly in Negroes or dark-skinned people.

siderosis Lung disease resulting from inhalation of iron dust.

sig. A prescription abbreviation for *signa*, meaning "label it."

sigmoid colon The S-shaped curve of the large bowel.

sigmoidectomy The surgical removal of the sigmoid portion of the large bowel.

sigmoiditis Inflammation of the sigmoid colon.

Simmond's disease A disease characterized by extreme emaciation and exhaustion.

simple fracture A bone break in which there is no break of the skin.

sinew Tendon.

singultus Hiccup.

sinistral A left-handed individual.

sinoatrial heart block A heart block due to interruption of normal impulses between the auricle and the point of origin of the normal heart beat.

sinus The hollow spaces in the bones surrounding the nose.

sinusitis Inflammation of one of the sinuses in the nose.

sinusotomy An operation to produce an artificial opening into a sinus, to allow pus to drain.

sinus rhythm The normal heart rhythm.

Sippy diet A 28-day diet composed mainly of milk and cream prescribed for some patients with peptic ulcer.

sister A registered nurse (British).

sitomania Excessive craving for food.

sitz bath A sitting bath, used to relieve pain and congestion in the rectal or pelvic areas.

skeleton The bones of the body.

Skene's glands The small mucous glands located on either side of the urethra.

skin The organ that envelops the body, composed of the dermis and epidermis.

skin grafting The transplantation of portions of the skin for cosmetic or medical purposes.

skin tabs Excessive skin around the anus often seen after the removal of hemorrhoids.

skull The bones that make up the head and the face.

sleeping sickness See *encephalitis*.

slough Dead tissue separating from living tissue.

smallpox A contagious infectious disease in which fever is followed by an eruption which produces scars.

smear Secretions of blood or tissue spread onto a glass slide for microscopical study.

smegma Ill-smelling secretions that sometimes accumulate under the foreskin and around the labia minora.

smoker's cancer A type of cancer of the lip observed in habitual smokers.

sodium bicarbonate Baking soda.

sodium bromide A chemical which tends to calm the nerves.

sodium chloride Salt.

sodomy Sexual intercourse by the anus, either between males, or with animals.

soft chancre Chancroid.

solar dermatitis A general term for skin eruptions caused by exposure to the sun.

solar plexus The nerve center in the upper abdomen containing nerves which supply the stomach, liver, and other organs.

soleus A flat muscle of the calf.

soluble Capable of dissolving.

solvent A liquid which can dissolve a substance.

soma The body.

somatic Pertaining to the body.

somatomegaly Gigantism.

somnambulism Sleepwalking.

somnambulist One who walks in his sleep.

somnifacient A drug producing sleep.

somniloquy Talking in one's sleep.

143

somnolism Hypnotism.

somnus Sleep.

Sonne dysentery A form of intestinal infection.

soporific Causing deep sleep.

sorbefacient An agent that aids absorption.

sore A wound.

sore throat Tonsillitis, laryngitis, pharyngitis—alone or in combination.

S.O.S. A prescription abbreviation for *si opus sit*, if necessary.

sound A long metal instrument inserted into a body channel in order to determine if the passageway is open.

Spanish fly See *cantharides*.

spasm A sudden involuntary muscular contraction.

spasmodic Pertaining to or characterized by spasms.

spasmophemia Stuttering.

spastic Marked by muscle spasms, usually recurrent.

speculum Any instrument for looking into a body cavity.

sperm The male germ cell.

spermatic cord The cord leading from the testicle to the seminal vesicle and carrying semen.

spermatocystitis Inflammation of the seminal vesicles.

spermatogenesis The process by which male sperm cells are formed.

spermatorrhea Involuntary discharge of semen (without orgasm).

spermaturia The presence of sperm in the urine.

spermicide A contraceptive which kills sperm on contact.

sphenoid The wedge-shaped bone at the base of the skull.

sphenoiditis Inflammation of the sphenoid sinus.

sphenoid sinus A cavity in the sphenoid bone behind and above the nose containing an outlet which drains into the nasal cavity.

spherocytosis An inherited disease in which the red blood cells rupture easily. Also known as *chronic familial jaundice* or *hemolytic anemia*.

sphincter A muscle surrounding and controlling the opening and closing of an opening.

sphincteralgia Pain in a sphincter muscle.

sphincterismus A painful muscle spasm involving the sphincter surrounding the anus.

sphincteritis Inflammation of the anal sphincter.

sphincter of Oddi The sphincter surrounding the end of the bile duct at the entrance to the small intestine.

sphincterotomy The surgical cutting of a sphincter.

sphygmomanometer An instrument for measuring blood pressure.

sphygmus The pulse.

spina bifida A birth deformity in which the vertebrae of the lower spine have failed to develop and close completely with the result that a hernia (rupture) occurs in which the spinal cord and nerves protrude through the back and appear beneath the skin.

spinal anesthesia Anesthesia produced by the injection of an anesthetic into the spinal area.

spinal canal The area, filled with spinal fluid, surrounding the spinal cord.

spinal cord That part of the central nervous system contained within the spinal column.

spinal fusion An operation for fusing vertebrae thereby making the spinal column rigid.

spinal hemiplegia Paralysis of one side of the body due to a lesion of the spinal cord.

spinal meningitis Inflammation of the meninges of the spinal cord.

spinal tap Lumbar puncture.

spine The backbone or spinal column.

spirochete Any spiral-shaped germ.

spleen A large, ductless organ in the upper left part of the abdomen.

splenectomy The surgical removal of the spleen.

splenitis Inflammation of the spleen.

splenocele Hernia or tumor of the spleen.

splenomegaly Enlargement of the spleen.

splint A support made of wood, metal, plaster, or other material for immobilizing the ends of a broken bone.

spondylarthritis Arthritis of the vertebrae.

spondylitis Inflammation of the vertebrae.

spondylolisthesis A deformity of the spine caused by the sliding forward of one vertebra.

spondylosis Fusion of the vertebrae.

spontaneous fracture A bone break occurring in bone diseases without injury.

spontaneous pneumothorax Air in the chest cavity and consequent lung collapse.

sporadic Occurring once in a while.

spotting A slight bloody discharge from the vagina not coming at the time it would normally be expected.

sprain The wrenching of a joint.

sprue A chronic nutritional deficiency disease marked primarily by fatty, "soapy" stools. Other symptoms include a sore mouth, a raw tongue, loss of weight, and weakness.

spur A pointed growth on a bone.

sputum Mucous material spit out of the mouth.

ss. A prescription abbreviation for *semis*, one-half.

stadium A period in the course of a disease.

stadium caloris The period of disease during which there is fever.

stadium sudoris The sweating stage of a disease.

stain A dye.

stalk A lengthy supporting part of tissue, as the stalk of a polyp.

stammer To speak haltingly.

Stanford-Binet test An intelligence test which is a revision of the Binet-Simon tests originally conducted in France by Binet and Simon.

stapedectomy An operation to restore lost hearing in which the stapes of the middle ear is removed and replaced with a prosthesis.

stapes The stirrup-shaped little bone of the middle ear.

staphylococcemia Blood poisoning caused by staphylococcus germs in the blood.

staphylococcus The general name for a group of ball-shaped bacteria which cause many human infections.

staphylorrhaphy The surgical repair of a cleft palate.

stasis The stoppage of normal flow of body fluids.

static At rest.

status anginosus A long lasting attack of angina pectoris.

status asthmaticus Continuous, unrelieved asthmatic attacks lasting from a few days to a week.

status epilepticus Attacks of epilepsy occurring one after another.

status lymphaticus Suffocation caused by enlargement of the thymus gland.

steatitis Inflammation of fat tissue.

steatoma A sebaceous cyst.

steatorrhea Fatty stools.

Steinmann pin A surgical nail, driven through the ends of bones in order to obtain traction in cases of fracture.

stenosis Narrowing of a body canal.

stercolith Very hard feces.

stercus Feces.

sterile Unable to have children; germ free.

sterility Inability to reproduce; an area in which no germs can live.

sterilize To make free from germs; to render incapable of procreation.

sterilizer An apparatus for making equipment free from germs.

sternal puncture Insertion of a hollow needle into the sternum to obtain bone marrow cells for diagnosis.

sternoclavicular Referring to both the collarbone and breastbone.

sternocleidomastoid The muscle of the neck that flexes the head.

sternocostal Pertaining to the sternum and ribs.

sternodynia Pain in the sternum.

sternomastoid Same as *sternocleidomastoid*.

sternotomy An operation in which the sternum is cut in order to gain access to the mediastinum.

sternum The breast-bone.

steroids Drugs of hormone origin.

stertorous respiration Snoring.

147

stethoscope An instrument used by physicians to listen to sounds heard in the body.

Stewart-Morel-Morgagni syndrome A condition characterized by overgrowth of the skull above the eye region, obesity and headache.

sthenia Normal vigor.

stigma Any mark on the skin.

stillbirth The birth of a dead child.

stillborn Born dead.

Still's disease A type of a chronic infectious arthritis in childhood.

stimulant A drug that stimulates some organ of the body to greater activity.

stimulus Anything that stimulates.

stitch Suture.

stoma A tiny opening in a surface.

stomach A pear-shaped sack of membrane-lined muscle, capable of holding two to three pints of food and processing for digestion.

stomach ache A popular term for any kind of abdominal pain.

stomachic A medication to stimulate the appetite.

stomach ulcer See *peptic ulcer*.

stomatalgia Pain in the mouth.

stomatitis Inflammation of the mucous membranes of the mouth.

stomatitis venenata Stomatitis caused by drugs.

stomatocace Ulcerative stomatitis.

stomatocatharsis Salivation.

stomatodynia Pain in the mouth.

stomatodysodia Foul breath.

stomatopathy Any disease of the mouth.

stomatorrhagia Copious bleeding from the mouth.

stomenorrhagia Bleeding in the mouth associated with abnormal menstruation.

stone A calcified solid.

stool Feces.

strabismus Squinting.

strabismus convergens Cross-eyedness in which one or both of the eyes turns in.

strabismus, divergent Crossed-eyes in which one or both of the eyes turn out.

strabotomy An operation to correct strabismus.

strain Pain in a muscle due to excessive stretching or overuse.

strangulated hernia An intestinal hernia in which circulation of the blood and feces are blocked.

strangulation Death caused by the inability to breathe because the air passage is blocked.

strangury Painful urination, with passage of urine drop by drop.

stratum A layer.

stratum spongiosum A spongy layer.

strawberry birthmark A birthmark looking like a strawberry, caused by dilated blood vessels in the skin.

streptococcemia Blood poisoning due to streptococci in the blood.

streptococcus A particular germ, sometimes called "strep," which may cause severe infections in humans.

streptomycin A powerful antibiotic drug useful against many germs.

stress In dentistry, the force exerted by the lower teeth against the upper during chewing.

stress incontinence Involuntary passing of urine upon sudden movement or physical effort.

striae Streaks or stripes.

striae cutis distensae White or gray, shiny stripes on the stomach skin, breasts or thighs, following prolonged stretching from pregnancy or obesity.

striated muscle Voluntary muscle, as in the arms and legs, composed of cross-striped muscle fibers.

stricture Any abnormal narrowing of a body organ.

stringent Binding.

stripping An operation for varicose veins in which large sections of the veins are removed with a metal "stripper."

stroke The sudden rupture or clotting of a blood vessel to the brain.

stroma The connective tissue of an organ.

stromuhr An instrument for measuring the speed of blood flow.

strongyloidiasis The Infection of the intestines with the *Strongyloides* roundworm.

struma A goiter.

stupefacient Narcotic.

stupefaction Stupor.

stupor Semiconsciousness.

stye An infection of a sebaceous gland of an eyelid.

styptic An agent that stops bleeding by causing contraction of the blood vessels.

subacute Inbetween acute and chronic.

subacute appendicitis Mild acute appendicitis.

subacute bacterial endocarditis An infection of the heart valves with *Streptococcus viridans*.

subarachnoid Underneath the middle membrane that covers the brain and spinal cord.

subarachnoid block A condition in which something prevents the normal flow of cerebrospinal fluid.

subarachnoid hemorrhage Hemorrhaging around the brain beneath the arachnoid membrane.

subarachnoid space The area beneath the arachnoid membrane.

subaxillary Under the armpit.

subclavian Beneath the collarbone.

subclinical Pertaining to a disease whose signs and symptoms are so mild that they go unnoticed.

subcostal Beneath the ribs.

subcutaneous Underneath the skin.

subcutaneous emphysema The accumulation of air underneath the skin.

subdelirium A mild delirium with lucid intervals.

subduct To draw downward.

subdural Beneath the membrane covering the brain and spinal cord.

subdural hematoma A blood clot within the skull lying beneath the outer covering of the brain, but on top of its inner covering.

subglossitis Inflammation of the tissue under the tongue.

subinvolution Imperfect return to normal size after an enlargement.

subinvolution of the uterus Failure of the uterus to return to its normal size after delivery.

subjacent Lying beneath.

sublethal Less than fatal.

sublingual Under the tongue.

subluxation An incomplete dislocation of a joint.

submandibular Underneath the lower jaw.

submaxillary Submandibular·

submaxillaritis Inflammation of a salivary gland.

submental Under the chin.

suboccipital Under the back of the head.

subordination The condition of organs that depend upon other organs.

subparalytic Incompletely paralytic.

subpectoral Located beneath the chest muscles.

subplantigrade Walking with the heel slightly elevated.

subpleural Situated beneath the membrane that covers the lungs.

subpleural bleb A blister on the outer surface of the lung just beneath the pleura.

subscapular Beneath the shoulder blade.

subserous Beneath a serous membrane.

substernal Beneath the breastbone.

substrate An underlayer; a substance upon which an enzyme acts.

subsultus Convulsive jerking.

subsultus tendinum A twitching of the muscles of the hands and feet accompanied by fever.

subtentorial Situated beneath the cerebellum.

sububeres Nursing children.

subungual Beneath a nail.

subvitaminosis A state of vitamin deficiency.

succorrhea An excessive flow of a secretion.

succus entericus Intestinal juice.

succus gastricus Stomach juice.

sucrose Sugar.

Sudeck's atrophy Degeneration of bone following injury.

sulfonamide drugs Drugs which are derived from sulfonamide.

sunburn A skin burn caused by the ultraviolet rays of the sun.

superego The conscience.

superficial Near the surface; not serious or profound.

suppository Any medication inserted into the rectum or vagina.

suppurate To form pus.

suppurative wound A wound from which pus is discharged.

surgeon A physician who is specially trained to perform operations.

suture To stitch an opening.

sweat glands Glands that release sweat through the skin.

sweat test A test for cystic fibrosis of the pancreas.

sycosis Inflammation of the hair roots.

Sydenham's chorea A disorder characterized by involuntary movements of the muscles of the face, arms and legs.

sympathectomy An operation in which the nerves of the sympathetic nervous system are cut; used for the relief of high blood pressure.

sympathetic nervous system The part of the nervous system which supplies and regulates most of the involuntary organs and muscles of the body.

sympathetic ophthalmia A severe inflammation of an eye, caused by an injury or disease of the other eye.

symptomatic treatment Treatment to relieve the patient's complaints rather than to cure the illness.

syncope Fainting.

syndrome A collection of symptoms which collectively characterize a disease.

synechia Adhesions of the iris to a neighboring part of the eye.

synergetic Pertaining to organs working together in harmony.

synergy The cooperative action of two or more organs.

synorchism Fusion of the two testicles.

synoscheos Joining of the skin of the penis with that of the scrotum.

synostosis The union of two or more bones which originally were separate.

synovectomy The surgical removal of the membrane of a joint.

synovial fluid The clear amber fluid found in various joints.

synovial membrane The thin lining membrane of a joint.

synovioendothelioma A malignant synovioma.

synovioma Any tumor originating in the membranes or sheaths of joints, tendons or bursae.

synovitis Inflammation of a joint lining membrane.

syphilid Any skin eruption due to syphilis.

syphilis A contagious venereal disease which can infect any of the body tissues.

syphilitic Having syphilis.

syphilitic cirrhosis Syphilis of the liver.

syphilitic node Localized swelling on bones due to syphilis.

syphiloma A tumor due to syphilis.

syphilophobia Abnormal fear of syphilis.

syringe An instrument used to inject fluid into the body.

systemic A condition or disease involving the entire body.

systole The phase of heart beat during which the heart contracts and expels the blood.

tabes Degeneration.

tabes dorsalis A degeneration of the nervous system caused by syphilis.

tabetic Pertaining to tabes.

tachycardia Rapid heart beat of more than 100 beats per minute.

tachypnea Abnormally rapid breathing.

tactile Referring to the sense of touch.

tacnia Tapeworms.

taint An inherited tendency toward development of a disease.

talalgia Pain in the ankle.

talipes Any one of a variety of deformities of the foot, espe cially *clubfoot*.

talipes planus Flatfoot.

talus Ankle bone, astragalus.

tampon A plug of cotton, or other absorbent material, introduced into a body cavity to stop bleeding or soak up secretions.

tannic acid An acid usually obtained from nutgall which, when applied to a burned area, tends to stop oozing and bleeding and forms a scab.

tapeworm Long, narrow flat worms which invade the intestinal tract.

tarantula A large spider whose bite is extremely painful but not fatal.

tarry stools Feces having the color and consistency of tar, usually due to hemorrhage in the intestinal tract.

tarsalgia Pain in the foot.

tarsometatarsal Referring to the bones of the foot.

tarsus The ankle.

tartar The hard deposits around the base of teeth.

tartar emetic A compound which induces spitting, nausea and vomiting.

Tay-Sach's disease Amaurotic familial idiocy. A progressive, fatal disease of infants associated with blindness and brain deterioration.

TB Tuberculosis.

teat A nipple.

technique The method of procedure.

tegmen A tissue covering.

telalgia Referred pain. Pain radiating to another part of the body.

telangiectasis Swelling and dilatation of capillaries sometimes resulting in a small tumor.

telangitis Inflammation of the capillaries.

telencephalon The front portion of the brain.

telepathy Awareness of the thoughts in another person's mind. Extrasensory perception.

154

temple The side of the head in front of and slightly above the ear.

temporal Referring to the region of the temple.

temporize To provide provisional treatment for a patient until a definitive diagnosis is established.

tender Painful to the touch.

tendon A band of connective tissue which attaches a muscle to another part of the body.

tendonitis Inflammation of a tendon.

tenesmus Straining to empty the bowels or to pass urine with resulting pain.

tenia A bandlike tissue.

tennis elbow Inflammation of a bursa in the elbow region.

tenophyte A bony or cartilage-type growth on a tendon.

tenoplasty Reparative surgery of a tendon.

tenorrhaphy An operation to repair torn tendons.

tenosynovitis Inflammation of a tendon and its sheath.

tenotomy Cutting or dividing a tendon for the correction of a deformity.

tenovaginitis Inflammation of the sheath of a tendon.

tension headache Muscle-contraction headache.

tensor A muscle that serves to make a part of the body tense.

tentative diagnosis A diagnosis subject to change when more is learned about the illness.

tentorium The tissue separating the cerebrum from the cerebellum in the brain.

tenuous Thin.

tepid Lukewarm.

teras A monster.

teratism A birth deformity.

teratocarcinoma A cancer tumor made of cell elements found in embryos.

teratoma Any tumor or new growth that includes embryonic tissue, especially teeth and hair of an unborn fetus that did not completely develop. Teratomas are most commonly found in the testicles and ovaries.

teratophobia Abnormal fear of monsters or deformed people.

terminal Referring to a patient who is about to die.

terramycin Trademark for a powerful antibiotic.

tertian Recurring every other day.

tertiary syphilis Syphilis which includes all of the symptoms of disease occurring after the fourth year of infection.

tertipara A woman who has given birth to three children.

testalgia Pain of the testicles.

testicle The male organ which produces sperm, located in the scrotum.

testicular Pertaining to the testicles.

testis A testicle.

test meal A type of food given to test the function of the stomach.

testosterone The male sex hormone.

tetanic Pertaining to tetanus.

test-tube babies Babies produced by artificial insemination.

tetanophobia An abnormal fear of tetanus.

tetanus Lockjaw. An infectious disease which especially attacks the muscles of the neck and lower jaw. The tetanus germ enters the body through a cut or injury and is associated with convulsions and severe muscle spasms.

tetanus toxoid Tetanus vaccine.

tetany A disease caused by insufficient calcium in the blood and accompanied by muscle spasms and convulsions. It is not related to tetanus.

tetralogy of Fallot A birth deformity of the heart.

texis Childbearing.

thalamus The part of the brain situated at the base of the brain, below the cerebrum.

thalamotomy The surgical destruction of parts of the thalamus, usually for the treatment of intractable pain.

thalassophobia A fear of the sea.

thamuria Frequent urination.

thanatoid Deathlike.

thanatology The study of death.

thanatophobia Fear of death.

thebaic Pertaining to opium.

theca A sheath.

thecitis Inflammation of the sheath of a tendon.

thelalgia Pain in a nipple.

thelasis Suckling a breast.

theleplasty Plastic surgery of the nipple.

thelerethism Erection of the nipple, brought on by stimulation or excitement.

thelitis Inflammation of a nipple.

thelium The nipple.

thenar The palm of the hand.

theomania A form of insanity in which the individual believes himself to be a godly being.

therapeusis Therapeutics.

therapeutic Curative.

therapeutic abortion Termination of a pregnancy.

therapeutics The branch of medical science dealing with the treatment of disease.

therapist One who treats an illness, disease or condition.

therapy Treatment of disease.

theriodic Malignant.

therioma A malignant tumor.

thermal Pertaining to heat.

thermoanesthesia The loss of the sense of heat.

thermocouple An instrument for measuring skin temperatures.

thermometer An instrument used to measure the temperature of the body.

thermophagy The habit of eating very hot food.

thermoplegia Sunstroke.

thermotherapy Treatment of disease by heat.

thiamine Part of the vitamin B complex.

Thiersch grafts Large, thin slices of skin which are transplanted onto large wounds in the hope that they will grow.

thigh The part of the leg from the pelvis to the knee.

thighbone The femur.

thiouracil A powerful drug containing sulfur.

third-degree burn A burn that destroys the skin and its underlying tissues.

Thomsen's disease The absence of muscle function and coordination due to a birth defect.

thoracectomy Cutting into the wall of the chest and removing all or part of a rib.

thoracocentesis Puncturing the chest wall, generally with a hollow needle, and withdrawing accumulated fluids from the chest cavity.

thoracic Pertaining to the chest.

thoracolumbar spine The parts of the spine from the chest down to the lower back.

thoracoplasty An operation for collapsing a lung by removing the ribs to which it adheres.

thoracotomy A surgical incision into the chest cavity, for diagnostic purposes or to carry out treatment.

thorax The chest.

Thorazine Trademark for *chlorpromazine*, a tranquilizer.

three-day measles Rubella.

threshold stimulus The smallest stimulus that produces response.

threshold pain The point at which pain can be felt.

throat The pharynx.

thrombectomy The surgical removal of a blood clot from a blood vessel.

thromboangiitis obliterans A chronic inflammatory disease of the arteries and veins.

thrombocyte A blood platelet.

thrombocytopenia A decrease in the number of red blood platelets which occurs in blood diseases such as purpura.

thromboembolism The blocking of a blood vessel by a dislodged clot in a distant blood vessel.

thrombolysis Breaking up of a blood clot within a vessel.

thrombophilia A tendency to form blood clots.

thrombophlebitis Inflammation of a vein accompanied by clot formation within that vein.

thrombose To clot.

thrombosis The formation of a blood clot.

thrombus A blood clot in a blood vessel which remains stationary.

thrush A fungus infection of the mouth in infants and occasionally older persons characterized by white patches on the tongue and membranes of the mouth.

thymic Referring to the thymus gland.

thymitis Inflammation of the thymus.

thymal turbidity test A test for liver disease.

thymus gland A gland located in the chest near the heart. The thymus is active during the first eight or nine months of life. After the second year, it normally shrinks almost to the point of disappearance and is replaced by other types of tissue.

thyreogenic Of thyroid origin.

thyroglossal cyst A cyst in the front of the neck composed of cells coming from the tongue and thyroid gland.

thyroid The thyroid gland.

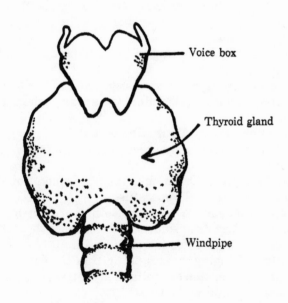

The thyroid gland.

thyroid crisis A severe, often fatal, condition stemming from extreme overactivity of the thyroid gland.

thyroidectomy The surgical removal of all or part of the thyroid gland.

thyroid gland One of the most important of the endocrine glands which lies in the front part of the throat alongside the windpipe.

thyroid heart disease Heart disease associated with changes of thyroid function.

thyroid hormone Thyroxine, liothyronine, or both.

thyroiditis Inflammation of the thyroid gland.

thyroid storm See *thyriodic crisis*.

thyromegaly Enlargement of the thyroid gland.

thyrotoxicosis Hyperthyroidism. Overactivity of the thyroid gland; goiter.

thyroxin A hormone manufactured by the thyroid gland.

tibia The larger of the two bones of the leg, commonly called the shinbone.

tibiofibular Pertaining to the tibia and fibula, the bones of the leg.

tic A twitching of muscles, especially of the face.

tic douloureux Trigeminal neuralgia; sharp pains in the face.

tick fever Rocky Mountain spotted fever.

t.i.d. A prescription abbreviation for *ter in die*, three times a day.

tidal drainage Draining urine from a non-functioning bladder with a special apparatus.

Tietze's disease A painful swelling of the rib cartilages.

tincture Any drug solution in alcohol.

tinea A fungus infection of the skin.

tinnitus Ringing, buzzing sounds in the ears.

tissue A collection of similar body cells such as muscle tissue, fat tissue, and nerve tissue.

titubation Loss of balance caused by a disease of the brain or spinal cord.

tobacosis Nicotine poisoning due to excessive smoking.

tocus; tokus Childbirth.

tolerance The ability to endure the influence of a drug or poison.

tongue The muscular organ connected to the floor of the back of the mouth whose chief functions are to help in chewing, swallowing, taste, and the formation of sounds in speech.

tongue-tie A birth deformity in which the tongue has an abnormally short band under it which binds it to the floor of the mouth making speech difficult.

tonsil Lymph glands located in the mouth near the back of the tongue.

tonsillectomy The surgical removal of the tonsils.

tonsillitis Inflammation of the tonsils.

tonus The normal degree of contraction present in muscles.

topalgia Localized pain without organic causes.

tophi Chalky stone deposits found in or near joints in gout.

topical Local.

toponeurosis A localized neurosis; an emotional disturbance surrounding a specific event.

torpid Sluggish.

torpor Sluggish inactivity.

torsion Twisting, the term describes the twisting of organs in the body thereby limiting their blood supply.

torso The trunk of the body.

torticollis A spasmodic movement of the neck muscles which causes the head to be pulled toward one side.

tortuous Containing many turns and twists.

torulosis Cryptococcosis, a yeast infection involving the brain, skin and lungs.

torniquet Any apparatus for controlling hemorrhage.

toxemia Poisonous products (toxins) in the blood.

toxemia of pregnancy A disease of pregnancy caused by poisons circulating in the blood. Symptoms include vomiting, elevated blood pressure, chronic nephritis, acute yellow atrophy of the liver, pre-eclampsia and eclampsia.

toxic Poisonous.

toxic hepatitis Inflammation of the liver caused by the action of poisonous compounds.

toxicity The degree to which a substance can poison the body.

toxicoderma A disease of the skin caused by poison.

toxicology The scientific study of poisons and their antidotes.

toxicosis Poisoning of the entire body.

toxic psychosis A brain disorder caused by a toxic agent such as alcohol or opium.

toxin A poison.

toxoplasmosis Infection with the parasite *Toxoplasma gondii*; usually encountered in infants, who may suffer repeated convulsions.

tr. A prescription abbreviation for *tinctura*, tincture.

trachea The windpipe.

tracheitis Inflammation of the trachea.

trachelectomy The surgical removal of the neck of the uterus.

trachelitis Inflammation of the neck of the uterus; cervicitis.

trachelodynia Pain in the neck.

trachelorrhaphy The surgical repair of a torn cervix.

tracheobronchial Referring to the trachea and bronchial tubes which extend from it.

tracheobronchitis Inflammation of the trachea and bronchial tubes.

tracheotomy Cutting into the windpipe from the front of the throat to provide a temporary air passage.

trachoma A highly contagious disease of the eyelids, caused by a virus; a form of conjunctivitis.

tracing A recording, such as is made of the heart in an electrocardiography.

tract A pathway; a bundle of nerve fibers; a group of parts or organs serving a special purpose.

traction Pulling, drawing or stretching. It usually means the setting of broken bones in which the limbs or head are pulled in a definite direction and kept that way by weights, pulleys and frames. Often used in back injuries.

trait Any characteristic of an individual.

trance The hypnotic state.

tranquilizer A drug given to calm the nerves.

transanimation Mouth-to-mouth resuscitation.

transect To cut across.

transection Cutting through, as of a bone in an amputation.

transfixion The piercing of a structure.

transformation A change in form, structure, or function.

transfusion The introduction into a blood vessel of blood, or some other liquid.

transfusion reaction A reaction caused by introducing blood which is incompatible with the blood of the recipient.

translucent Partially transparent.

transmission The transfer of infectious disease from one person to another.

transpiration The transfer of fluid through the skin.

transplant A tissue or organ taken from one part of the body and implanted in another part of the body or in another person.

transplantation Any operation involving a transplant or grafting.

transplantation immunity The rejection of a transplanted tissue or organ by the body's defense mechanisms.

transurethral prostatectomy The surgical removal of the prostate through the penis using an operating cystoscope.

transvaginal Through the vagina.

transverse Crosswise.

transverse colon The portion of the large bowel which lies across the upper abdomen.

transverse lie When the baby emerges by the shoulders, one arm appearing first during childbirth.

transvestism Dressing in the clothing of the opposite sex.

trapezius The large muscle stretching over the shoulder from the back of the neck to the collarbone which elevates the shoulder.

trauma An injury caused by an outside force.

traumatic Caused by a wound or injury.

trembling Quivering.

tremor Involuntary shaking, or quivering.

tremulous Trembling.

trench foot Frostbite of the foot.

trench mouth Inflammation of the gums with ulcers that may also extend to the tonsils (*Vincent's angina*).

trepanning An operation in which a hole is bored in the skull.

trepidation Anxiety.

Treponema pallidum The germ that causes syphilis.

triad A group of three signs and symptoms, indicating a specific disease.

triage Sorting out the wounded so that the most serious cases can be treated first.

tribade A woman who plays the role of the male in a lesbian relationship.

triceps The muscles in the back of the upper arms which extend the elbow.

trichinosis A parasitic disease caused by eating infected pork which affects muscles and causes nausea, vomiting, dizziness and diarrhea.

trichitis Inflammation at the roots of the hair.

trichobezoar A tuft of hair in the stomach or bowels sometimes seen in mentally ill patients who eat their own hair.

trichoid Resembling hair.

trichomonas vaginitis Vaginitis caused by an accompanied discharge and irritation. The condition can be treated with antibiotics, but may recur.

trichomycosis A fungus infection of the hair.

trichophagy Eating hair.

trichophytosis Fungus infection of the scalp, face, beard, body, crotch or nails.

trichuriasis Invasion by roundworms.

trifacial nerve The trigeminal nerve.

trifocal lenses Eyeglasses for near, intermediate, and far vision.

trigeminal nerve The fifth cranial nerve, supplying the face.

trigeminal neuralgia Sharp pains in the face, along the course of the trigeminal nerve. Tic douloureux.

trigger action A sudden stimulus that initiates a process that may have nothing in common with the action that started it.

trigonitis Inflammation of the bladder; a form of cystitis.

triorchid An individual having three testicles.

tripara A woman who has borne three children.

triplegia Hemiplegia with the additional paralysis of one limb on the opposite side.

trismus Severe spasm of the muscles of the jaw; tetanus.

trisomy 21 syndrome Down's syndrome.

trocar A surgical instrument with a sharp point, used to remove fluids.

troche A lozenge.

tromomania Delirium tremens.

trophic Pertaining to nutrition.

trophoneurosis Any disease caused by a disturbance of the nerves which are connected to the diseased region.

tropical anhidrotic asthenia Heat exhaustion caused by an inability to sweat.

tropical disease A disease encountered in the tropics.

true ribs The seven upper ribs on each side that are attached to the sternum.

true skin The dermis or lower layer of the skin.

truncated Shortened.

trunk The torso; the body without head or limbs.

truss A support worn to hold a hernia in place.

trypanosomiasis Sleeping sickness, caused by infestation of the blood by the *trypanosome*.

trypsin An intestinal enzyme which breaks down proteins.

tsp An abbreviation for teaspoonful.

tsutsugomushi disease A disease characterized by headache, high fever, and a rash, occurring in the Far East. This is a rickettsial disease transmitted by the bite of an infected insect.

tubal pregnancy Pregnancy taking place in the fallopian tubes.

tubercle A small nodule; a rounded lump on a bone; the inflammatory reaction caused by the tuberculosis germ.

tubercular Having many tubercles.

tuberculin test A skin test to determine the presence of tuberculosis.

tuberculosis Any infection caused by *Mycobacterium tuberculosis*. Infection of the lungs.

tuberculous Infected with tuberculosis.

tuberosity A part of a bone that protrudes.

tuboplasty   The repair of a fallopian tube using plastic.

tubule   A small tube.

tularemia   Rabbit fever; an infectious disease transmitted to man by infected animals, or through an insect bite.

tumescence   A swelling.

tumor   An abnormal growth of useless cells anywhere in the body.

tumorous   Having the characteristics of a tumor.

tunic   A membrane covering an organ.

tunica vaginalis   The membranes covering the testicles.

turbid   Cloudy.

turgid   Swollen; congested.

twilight sleep   Partial anesthesia during childbirth.

twin   One of a pair born at the same time.

twin, fraternal   Twins originating from two separate eggs and therefore not necessarily of the same sex or appearance.

twin, identical   Twins originating from a single egg which are therefore identical in every way.

twin, Siamese   Twins joined one to the other at some part of their bodies.

tympanic membrane   The eardrum.

tympanites   Distention of the abdomen due to excessive gas in the intestines.

tympanitis   Inflammation of the middle ear and eardrum.

tympanoplasty   An operation to repair a damaged eardrum.

typhoid fever   An infection caused by the typhoid bacillus resulting in high fever, ulcers of the intestine, diarrhea, headache, weakness, and hemorrhages.

typhus fever   An infectious disease caused by a rickettsial organism often transmitted by the bite of infected body lice. It has no relation to typhoid fever. It is characterized by high fever, headache, a body rash, mental confusion. Recovery takes about two weeks.

typical   Following the usual pattern.

uberty   Fertility.

ulcer   Any open sore with an inflamed base the result of the destruction of skin or mucous membrane, with or without infection or pain. As the tissue disintegrates it leaves a running sore. Ulcers can occur on any part of the skin or mucous linings.

ulcerate To form an ulcer.

ulcerative colitis A form of colitis associated with diarrhea, ulcerations of the large bowel, pain, and rectal bleeding.

ulcerogenic Tending to produce ulcers.

ulcus An ulcer.

ulitis Inflammation of the gums; gingivitis.

ulna The long bone of the inside of the forearm. The other bone of the forearm is the *radius*.

ulocace Ulcerative inflammation of the gums.

uloid Scar-like.

ulorrhagia Bleeding from the gums.

ultraviolet radiation Light rays that occur beyond the violet end of the visible spectrum. Sunlight is an example.

umbilical cord The cord connecting the unborn child with the placenta.

umbilicus The navel.

unciform Hook-shaped.

uncinariasis Hookworm invasion.

unconscious In a coma-like state.

unction An ointment.

undescended testicle A testicle which has not come down into the scrotum.

undinism Sexual excitement aroused by passing urine.

undulant fever Malta fever. An infection from the brucella germ often caused by drinking unpasteurized milk or by contact with infected animals. Symptoms generally include aches and pains, headache, sweating, and a prolonged fever.

ungual Pertaining to the nails.

unigravida A woman who is pregnant for the first time.

unilateral On one side only.

union Growing together into one.

United States Pharmacopeia The official U.S. publication listing all drugs and medications. Abbreviated *U.S.P.*

United States Public Health Service The federal agency concerned with the development of a public health program within the jurisdiction of the federal government.

universal donor   A blood donor of group "O" which all recipients can accept.

universal recipient   An individual of the AB blood group.

Unna's paste boot   A casing for the leg used in treating varicose ulcers and veins made by applying a medicated paste to the leg. A bandage is then placed over the paste.

upside-down stomach   A protrusion of the stomach up through the diaphragm and into the lungs.

uracrasia   Inability to control the flow of urine.

uraniscus   The palate.

uranism   Homosexuality.

uranoplasty   An operation to repair a cleft palate in the roof of the mouth.

urea   A compound found in the blood and urine.

uremia   An illness caused by the inability of the kidneys to eliminate waste products of metabolism with the resulting build-up of an excess of urea.

uresis   Urination.

ureter   Either of the tubes through which urine passes from the kidneys into the bladder.

ureteritis   Inflammation of a ureter.

ureterolithiasis   A stone in the ureter.

ureterolithotomy   Surgical removal of a stone from a ureter.

ureteromegaly   Abnormal enlargement of the ureter.

ureterorrhagia   Bleeding from a ureter.

ureterotomy   A surgical incision of a ureter.

uretero-ureterostomy   An operation in which a ureter from one kidney is sutured to the ureter of the other kidney.

urethra   The mucus-lined tube that carries urine from the bladder outside the body.

urethritis   Inflammation of the urethra, usually the result of infection, but also from other causes.

urethroplasty   An operation on the urethra.

urethroscope   An illuminated instrument for examining the inside of the urethra.

urinalysis   Examination of the urine for chemical composition.

urine The watery fluid excreted by the kidneys, stored in the bladder, and discharged through the urethra.

urinoma A cyst containing urine.

urning A male homosexual.

urochesia Discharge of urine through the anus.

uroclepsia Involuntary or unconscious urination.

urogenital Pertaining to the organs of reproduction and urination; genitourinary.

urography X-ray pictures of the urinary tract, taken with dyes.

urologist A physician who specializes in diseases of the urogenital system.

urorrhagia Excessive discharge of urine, as in diabetes insipidus.

urticaria An allergic condition of the skin characterized by the formation of large welts which itch a great deal. Also known as hives.

urticaria solaris Urticaria caused by exposure to sunlight.

U.S.P. Abbreviation for United States Pharmacopeia.

USPHS Abbreviation for United States Public Health Service.

uteralgia Pain in the womb.

uterine Pertaining to the uterus.

uterine tubes Fallopian tubes.

uterogestation Normal pregnancy.

uterometer An instrument used to measure the womb.

uteropelvic Pertaining to the womb and the ligaments which hold it in place.

uterovaginal Pertaining to the uterus and vagina.

uterus The female organ in which the embryo develops; the womb.

uterus bicornis A womb which has not developed fully and has two parts, or horns.

uterus didelphys A uterus divided into two compartments caused by a failure to join during development.

uvea The pigmented layer of the eye, including iris, ciliary body and choroid.

uveitis Inflammation of the uvea of the eye.

uvula The conical piece of muscle tissue which hangs down from the soft palate in the back of the mouth. In some throat conditions it may become elongated and hang down so far that it brushes against the tongue.

uvulectomy Surgical removal of an elongated uvula.

uvulitis Inflammation of the uvula.

uvulotomy Cutting off the uvula surgically.

vaccinate To immunize against a disease.

vaccination Inoculation with a preparation containing disease germs·in order to prevent diseases caused by these organisms.

vaccine Any material administered to protect against germ invasion. The term is usually applied to preparations of virus or bacteria which will build up body resistance against the bacteria when injected into the body.

vaccinia A virus disease of cattle which, when used to inoculate man, induces immunity to smallpox.

vaccinophobia Fear of vaccination.

vacuum A space from which all air has been withdrawn.

vagabondage An uncontrollable desire to wander from home.

vagina Birth canal and female organ of sexual intercourse.

vaginal Pertaining to the vagina.

vaginal discharge A mucous discharge which may occur from the fourth week of pregnancy onward.

vaginal smear "Pap" smear. A diagnostic test to discover cancer.

vaginismus A painful spasm of the vagina due to contraction of the vaginal walls, thereby preventing intercourse.

vaginitis Inflammation of the vagina.

vaginomycosis A fungus infection of the vagina.

vaginoplasty The surgical repair of a torn vagina.

vagitus The cry of an infant.

vagotomy An operation to cut the vagus nerve.

vagus nerve The tenth and largest cranial nerve, serving the heart, lungs and the abdominal organs.

valetudinarian An invalid.

valgus Turned outward. The term is applied to clubfoot (talipes valgus), knock-knees (genu valgum), and out-of-line hips (coxa valga).

Valium Trademark for *diazepam*, a tranquilizer.

Valsalva's maneuver Blowing out a collapsed eustachian tube by closing the mouth and nose, and then forcefully expelling air from the lungs.

valve A mechanism which permits the contents to pass through but which prevents backflow. The heart and many other parts of the body contain valves.

valvotomy A surgical incision into a valve.

valvular Pertaining to a valve.

valvulectomy The surgical removal of a valve.

valvulitis Inflammation of a valve, usually of the heart.

valvulotomy The surgical removal of a heart valve to relieve constriction.

vapor bath A bath in which the bather is exposed to moist vapors.

varicella Chickenpox.

varices Dilated or swollen veins.

varicocele A swelling of the veins in the spermatic cord forming a soft often uncomfortable swelling.

varicocelectomy The surgical removal of a varicocele with or without removal of a part of the scrotum. This is a serious operation performed only when the veins are very large and the patient is in pain.

varicophlebitis Inflammation of a varicose vein.

varicose veins Veins that have become abnormally dilated and twisted.

varicotomy The surgical removal of a varicose vein.

variola Smallpox.

varix A varicose vein.

varus Turned inward; the opposite of valgus.

vas A vessel.

vas deferens The tube which conveys sperm from the testicles to the glands where they are stored ready for ejaculation.

vascular Relating to blood vessels.

vascular bed The entire blood supply of a part of the body.

vasectomy An operation for sterilizing the male by cutting through or removing part of the vas deferens.

vasitis Inflammation of the vas deferens.

Vaseline A trademark for a petroleum jelly.

vasoconstriction The narrowing and contraction of blood vessels.

vasodepressor A medication that lowers the blood pressure.

vasodilatation Enlargement of blood vessels.

vasomotor Controlling the dilatation of blood vessels. *Vasomotor nerves* are small peripheral nerves attached to the walls of blood vessels.

vasomotor reflex Constriction of a blood vessel in response to stimulation.

vasomotor rhinitis Allergic rhinitis.

vasomotor system The nerve supply of the blood vessels.

vasopressor Any substance which causes constriction of blood vessels and a rise in blood pressure.

VD Abbreviation for venereal disease.

vector A form of animal life which carries germs from a sick person to a healthy person.

vehicle A substance used as a mixer with an active drug.

vein stripper A long-handled, ring-tipped surgical instrument, used to remove varicose veins.

veins Blood vessels leading to the heart.

vellicate To twitch.

vena cava The two large veins that empty directly into the heart.

venectomy The surgical excision of all or part of a vein.

venereal disease Disease acquired principally through sexual intercourse, such as syphilis or gonorrhea.

venereal sore Chancre.

venereal ulcer Chancroid.

venereophobia Abnormal fear of getting a venereal disease.

venery Sexual intercourse.

venesection Blood-letting; cutting into a vein to draw out blood.

venipuncture Inserting a needle into a vein.

venogram X-ray of a vein.

venom Poison secreted by reptiles and insects.

venous Pertaining to the veins.

venter The belly; the abdomen.

ventral Referring to the stomach-side; the opposite of dorsal, back-side.

ventral hernia A hernia in which there is a protrusion through the abdominal wall.

ventricle A cavity such as the left and right ventricles of the heart, and the ventricles of the brain.

ventricular Referring to a ventricle.

ventricular fibrillation A heart irregularity originating in the ventricles.

ventricular puncture The insertion of a hollow needle into one of the ventricles of the brain.

ventricular septal defect An abnormal opening between the left and right ventricles of the heart.

ventriculitis Inflammation of the lining of the ventricles of the brain.

ventriculoatrial shunt An operation on the brain for the relief of hydrocephaly.

ventriculogram An x-ray picture of the ventricles of the brain.

ventriculoscopy Examination of the ventricles of the brain with an endoscope.

venule A small vein.

vermicide A medicine which kills worms.

vermifuge A medication that kills or expels intestinal worms.

vermin Lice.

vernal conjunctivitis A form of conjunctivitis recurring each spring or summer and disappearing with frost.

verruca Wart.

version Changing the position of the fetus in the womb in the course of childbirth so that it will be more safely and easily delivered.

vertebra One of the bones forming the spinal column.

vertebral Pertaining to a vertebra.

vertebral canal The canal which contains the spinal cord and its meninges.

vertebrectomy The surgical removal of a portion of a vertebra.

vertex The top of the skull.

vertex presentation The most common childbirth position (with the back of the head first).

vertigo Loss of spatial perspective.

vesical Pertaining to the urinary bladder.

vesicant Anything that produces blisters.

vesicle A small blister.

vesicotomy A surgical cut in the urinary bladder; a cystotomy.

vesiculitis Inflammation of the glands at the base of the prostate which store semen.

viable Able to live; a term applied to an embryo in the womb.

vibrio Germs shaped like short, curved rods.

vibrissae The hairs in the nose.

vicarious menstruation The discharge of blood from some other part of the body than the vagina during menstruation.

Vincent's angina Trench mouth; an infection of the mouth and throat due to a spiral organism.

viral Caused by a virus.

viremia Infection of the blood stream with a virus.

virile Masculine.

virilism The development of physical male characteristics in the female.

virulence Infectiousness; the disease-producing power of a germ.

virus A tiny organism capable of causing various infectious or contagious diseases.

viscera The internal organs of the abdomen and chest.

visceroptosis Sagging of the intestines and other organs of the abdomen.

viscid Sticky; thick.

viscous Semifluid.

viscus Any internal organ, such as the stomach or intestines.

vis medicatrix naturae The healing power of nature.

visual Pertaining to sight.

visus Vision.

vital Pertaining to life.

vitamins Substances found in foods in minute quantities which are needed for the normal functioning of the body. Deficiencies may cause diseases such as beri-beri, scurvy, pellagra, and rickets.

vitiligo A pigmentary disorder in which the coloring matter disappears in spots from the skin. These spots then appear white, in contrast to the normal coloration of the rest of the skin.

vitreous Glassy.

vitreous humor The jellylike transparent fluid filling the inside of the eyeball.

vivisection Surgery upon animals for the purpose of research.

vocal cords The two cords of tissue in the throat which make speech possible.

void To pass urine.

vola The palm of the hand or the sole of the foot.

volitional Voluntary.

volvulus A twist of the bowel around itself.

vomer The thin plate of bone that divides the nose into two nostrils.

vomiting The expelling of the contents of the stomach through the mouth.

vomiturition Retching.

vomitus cruentes Bloody vomit.

vomitus merinus Seasickness.

vomitus matutinus Morning sickness.

von Recklinghausen's disease A disease characterized by the formation of small tumors along the course of certain nerves.

voracious Having an abnormal appetite.

vox The voice.

voyeur A person who obtains sexual gratification from watching others perform sex acts or from viewing persons in the nude.

vulvar anus An abnormal condition in which the rectum opens into the vulva.

vulvectomy An operation for the removal of all or parts of the vulva.

vulvitis Inflammation of the vulva.

vulvovaginitis Inflammation of both the vulva and the vagina.

walleye A condition in which one or both eyes are off center and point in an outward direction.

ward A large hospital room in which there are several patients.

warts Growths on the skin.

Wassermann test A test used to determine whether or not a person has syphilis.

water on the brain A nonmedical term for *hydrocephalus*.

wean To discontinue breast feeding.

webbed fingers (or toes) A birth deformity in which a thin membrane connects two or more fingers or toes.

Well's disease A severe type of jaundice caused by infection with a spirochete germ.

wen A small cyst involving the oil glands of the skin.

Wertheim operation The surgical removal of the entire uterus, including the tubes, ovaries, ligaments and tissues surrounding them.

wet brain Edema of the brain.

wet nurse A woman who breast feeds an infant not her own.

wheal A swollen, itching area on the skin.

wheeze A whistling cough.

whiplash injury A sprain of the muscles and tendons of the back of the neck, caused by a sudden back jerk of the head.

Whipple's disease A generalized disease in which the lining and absorptive channels of the intestines become filled with fat.

whitlow Finger-tip infection.

WHO Abbreviation for *World Health Organization*.

whooping cough A serious childhood disease characterized by a convulsive cough, and affecting the mucous membrane of the respiratory system. The cough leaves the patient out of breath and the deep breathing resulting produces the whooping sound.

Widal test A blood test for typhoid fever.

Wilm's tumor A malignant growth that affects the kidneys of children, usually under six years of age.

windpipe Trachea.

winter cough Chronic bronchitis recurring every winter.

wisdom tooth The third molar tooth.

witch's milk Milk sometimes secreted from the breasts of a newborn baby.

withdrawal The interruption of intercourse before climax; *coitus interruptus*.

womb The uterus.

World Health Organization An agency of the United Nations whose purpose is to assist governments in the field of health.

wrist The link joining the forearm and the hand.

writer's cramp Spasm of the muscles of the hand and arm in people who do a lot of writing.

wryneck A twisted neck; torticollis.

xanthelasma A benign, yellow-colored, flat growth on the eyelids.

xanthocyanopia A vision defect in which yellow and blue colors are perceived, while red and green colors are not.

xanthoma A flat yellow tumor which may develop on the surface of the skin caused by a deposit of a fatty substance.

xanthomatosis A deposit of yellow-colored cells throughout the tissues and organs of the body.

xanthopsia Yellow vision; the condition in which objects look yellow, sometimes occurring in jaundice.

xanthosis A yellowish discoloration of the skin, sometimes seen in diabetes.

X chromosome A sex-determining gene found in the male sperm.

xenophobia A fear of strangers.

xeroderma A disorder in which the skin becomes rough, dry, and sometimes discolored, with fine scaly shedding.

xeromenia Having all the symptoms of menstruation without any actual flow of blood.

xeromycteria Lack of moisture in the nose.

xerophthalmia A thickening of the conjunctiva of the eye due to vitamin A deficiency.

xerosis Abnormal dryness of a tissue such as the skin or mucous membranes.

xiphoid The lower end of the breast-bone.

X-rays Light rays which can penetrate through body tissues.

yaws A tropical infection caused by a germ related to that of syphilis. It is not a venereal disease. It is characterized by raspberry-colored growths on various parts of the body, especially the face, feet, legs, hands, and external genitals. The growths may join to form large masses and may become ulcerated.

Y chromosome A sex-determining gene found in the male sperm.

yellow baby A newborn infant with jaundice, suffering from *erythroblastosis fetalis*.

yellow fever An infectious disease caused by a virus which is transmitted by the bite of an infected mosquito. It is characterized by chills, fever, aches and pains, jaundice, black vomit, internal bleeding, kidney damage, uremia and, in many cases, death.

yellow jack Yellow fever.

yellow jaundice Same as jaundice.

zinc oxide A medication which relieves many skin irritations.

zona Shingles; herpes zoster.

zone A region; an area.

zonesthesia The feeling of being held in by a tight girdle.

zonule A small band.

zooerastia Sexual intercourse with an animal.

zoonoses Animal diseases that can be transmitted to man.

There are about 80 such diseases including rabies, bovine tuberculosis, and undulant fever.

zoophilism Extraordinary love of animals; sexual pleasure from stroking or fondling animals.

zoophobia A fear of animals.

zoopsia An hallucination of being chased by animals.

zoster Herpes zoster; shingles.

zygoma The cheekbone.

zygomatic Pertaining to the cheek region.

zygote The fertilized egg cell.

zymosis A condition caused by infection.